An Introduction to Physical Methods of Treatment in Psychiatry

Peter Dally
MB, FRCP, FRCPsych, DPM
Consultant Psychiatrist, Department of Psychological Medicine, Westminster Hospital, London

Joseph Connolly
MB, MPhil, MRCP, MRCPsych, DPM
Senior Lecturer in Psychiatry, Westminster Hospital Medical School, London; Honorary Consultant in Psychiatry, Westminster Hospital and Queen Mary's Hospital, London

SIXTH EDITION

Fifth and previous editions by
William Sargant and *Eliot Slater*

CHURCHILL LIVINGSTONE
EDINBURGH LONDON MELBOURNE AND NEW YORK 1981

CHURCHILL LIVINGSTONE
Medical Division of Longman Group Limited

Distributed in the United States of America by Churchill Livingstone Inc., 19 West 44th Street, New York, N.Y. 10036, and by associated companies, branches and representatives throughout the world.

Sixth edition 1981

Fifth and previous editions by
William Sargant and *Eliot Slater*

ISBN 0 443 02019 1

British Library Cataloguing in Publication Data
Dally, Peter
An introduction to physical methods of treatment in psychiatry. – 6th ed.
1. physical therapy 2. Psychiatry
I. Title II. Connolly, Joseph
III. Sargant, William
616.89′13 RC482 80–41298

Printed in Singapore by Kyodo Shing Loong Printing Industries Pte Ltd

An Introduction to Physical Methods of Treatment in Psychiatry

Preface

There has been a steady improvement of treatment in psychiatry during the past 8 years, since the last edition of the book appeared. This has also been a period of reassessment. The overenthusiastic claims for this or that drug or treatment have been exposed and replaced in some instances by nihilistic, 'anti-psychiatry' attitudes. Even so well established a treatment as e.c.t. has met with considerable criticisms, and not only from the ill-informed. Yet this has produced at least one useful result for practising psychiatrists. They have had to re-examine carefully their techniques, assess the value of their treatments, strip away the nonspecific placebo effects and see anew the specific nature of what their treatments actually achieve, and how useful these really are.

It is clear that psychotropic drugs, e.c.t., and psychosurgery all have specific therapeutic effects and disadvantages. It is apparent that these treatments are sometimes misused, prescribed unnecessarily, or for the wrong conditions, or withheld when the patient's symptoms might be rapidly lifted. There have been great changes in our detailed knowledge of this over the past 15 years. Antidepressant drugs, to take an example, have removed much of the past need for e.c.t., but they have not totally replaced it. E.c.t. is still needed in severe depression and in cases otherwise refractory to treatment. We still meet patients who have been given e.c.t. when they would have responded better, say, to a MAOI, and who now complain bitterly of memory upset. But even more common is the patient who has partially recovered with antidepressant drugs, and is allowed to drift for months, when a few e.c.t. would lift him into full recovery.

As a result of reassessing individual treatments we now have increased understanding and greater acceptance of the synergistic effect of treatments. Psychotherapists now recognise that a drug may allow them to make contact with patients otherwise inaccessible to them, and enable patients to make greater use of their psychotherapeutic insights. Behaviour therapy may not begin to show results until drugs have reduced a patient's anxiety to a tolerable level. Psychotherapists and behaviour therapists have begun to recognise that there are factors common to both their techniques, and that one is not altogether dissimilar from the other.

Although this book is essentially a description of physical methods of treatment, we hope that no one will overlook the need to take a broad view of treatment, to remove causes when these are removable, and to encourage a patient to develop wider, more resilient attitudes. Because of the emphasis in recent years on behaviour therapy, we have thought it politic to include a short chapter on this subject. We have also added chapters on sexual dysfunction and deviations, and on psychiatric disorders of women and of old age.

We have omitted the chapter on epilepsy. The subject may have merited a place in the earlier editions, especially as e.c.t. was then sometimes given in an attempt to regulate the epileptic's fits, and allow him to have them under ideal conditions. Modern antiepileptic treatment has outmoded such methods. Temporal lobe epilepsy is occasionally associated with schizophrenic-like behaviour, or with aggressive outbursts. Post-e.c.t. automatism may occasionally intrude in a differential diagnosis. Nonetheless, the treatment of such conditions is generally best left to neurologists and physicians more experienced in epilepsy than the average psychiatrist.

We have also left out the previous editions' chapters on insulin, both deep and modified. Deep insulin therapy no longer has any place in the treatment of schizophrenia. Modified insulin is rarely used, and then largely for its nonspecific effects. Weight can be increased more readily by means of other safer drugs, especially chlorpromazine.

In other respects we have generally followed the path of the earlier editions. Above all, we hope that we have conveyed in this edition the enthusiasm and dedication of the original authors, and especially their principle of 'therapeutic persistence'.

1981

P.D.
J.C.

Acknowledgements

We are grateful to Dr Joan Gomez for her advice and criticism, particularly on the subject of alcoholism, to Dr Ann Dally and, most of all, to Anne Lingham for the work she put into typing the book, and her ability to keep us sane.

We also wish to thank William Heinemann Medical Books Ltd. for permission to reproduce material from *Anorexia Nervosa* by Dally, Gomez and Isaacs, 1979.

1981

P.D.
J.C.

Contents

1. Psychotropic drugs 1
2. Electro-convulsion therapy 51
3. Psychosurgery 67
4. Psychotherapy and the use of drugs: narcoanalysis and abreaction 77
5. Behavioural psychotherapy 85
6. Psychosomatic medicine 96
7. Weight problems: treatment of anorexia, anorexia nervosa and obesity 103
8. Treatment of sexual dysfunction and deviation 127
9. Psychiatric disorders in women 132
10. Psychiatric disorders in old age 138
11. Treatment of alcoholic and other addictions 143
12. Child psychiatry 157

Index 163

1

Psychotropic drugs

PART 1. PRINCIPLES

Just as e.c.t., introduced in 1939, revolutionised the treatment of endogenous depressive illness, so the arrival of psychotropic drugs from the 1950s onwards profoundly changed the treatment of psychiatric disorders. Reserpine appeared in 1952, to be almost at once superseded by chlorpromazine, the first of the phenothiazine derivatives. Within a few years chlorpromazine became the standard treatment of schizophrenia, making deep insulin therapy (DIT) a matter of historical interest. Antidepressant drugs were introduced in 1957; they were found to alleviate depressive symptoms, unlike the amphetamines which merely produce a short-lived and sometimes uncomfortable arousal. Chlordiazepoxide, quickly followed by other benzodiazepine derivatives, became available in 1960. Understandably, in view of their safety and low dependence potential, these tranquillisers have largely replaced barbiturates and meprobamate in the treatment of anxiety states.

In addition to their direct therapeutic effects, psychotropic drugs have had other influences. Mental illness, now that it is more amenable to treatment, is more comprehensible, and therefore more acceptable to the general public. Patients in the UK are less likely to be incarcerated in vast, isolated mental hospitals. Today they are treated as outpatients, in day hospitals and centres, or if needing admission, in psychiatric units attached to general hospitals located near their families and friends. Locked hospital wards—except in special security units—are virtually a phenomenon of the past. Institutionalisation is less common. Patients are now part of a therapeutic community; they participate in group meetings, discuss their problems openly and realistically, engage in occupational therapy (OT), and steadily rebuild their self confidence in preparation for returning to the everyday world.

It is true that the concept of the therapeutic community was taking shape even before psychotropic drugs came on the scene. But it was their beneficial effects on patients, particularly in reducing disruptive and often destructive behaviour, that allowed these humane ideas to be put so widely into practice. On an individual level, many other treatments became effective as drugs broke the vicious circle created by anxiety and depression. Psychotherapy, individual or group, which previously had been ineffectual because of the patient's crippling tension and impulsive acting out, could now be utilised by him. Thus, by enlarging the therapeutic armamentarium, psychotropic drugs and physical treatments also created an atmosphere which enhanced their own efficacy.

Inevitably, psychotropic drugs have been abused. It has taken many years to begin to understand how these drugs work, when they should be prescribed and why, their effective dosage, and for how long they should be given. This applies especially to the tranquillisers, both minor and major varieties, and antidepressant drugs. By no means all schizophrenic patients for example, need a maintenance dose of a phenothiazine; yet many are still unnecessarily, even harmfully, prescribed them. Anxious and depressed patients are often given drugs routinely, when they should in fact be advised to face and deal with their problems. By all means give a tranquilliser when anxiety is such that the patient is incapable of tackling his problems, but never forget or ignore the underlying causes. Very few psychiatric disorders arise that are not the result of adverse external events interacting with a patient's constitutional make up. Of course, many patients may be unable to alter their circumstances; in which case a drug is necessary to help them adapt to or accept their unhappy situations.

It is plain therefore that every doctor prescribing a psychotropic drug must know why he is doing so, and what he expects. So too should a patient know the reasoning behind his treatment. Clearly a doctor cannot prescribe rationally until he has made a diagnosis and understood the main causes of his patient's distress. Only then can he assess the need for treatment, its nature, and for how long it may be required.

As well as the therapeutic effect of any drug he employs, he must know the likely side effects, dangers from idiosyncratic reactions, and ways in which it may interact with other drugs. He must always balance the probable good against the possible dangers of a treatment. Once a drug is prescribed, the doctor must be perceptive about his patient's reactions, be prepared to vary the dosage up or down, or to stop the drug if need be; for instance, if the patient becomes pregnant or develops heart, renal or liver failure, with consequent impairment of the drug's metabolism and excretion.

Today, armed with drugs that are therapeutically potent, it is apparent to doctors that many treatments given in the past had no specific effects. Rather, they worked because of their placebo and nonspecific qualities, because the doctor wanted them to help, and because the patient needed to believe in them. Placebo effects have long been recognised and utilised; shape, size and colour of a drug, and dosage schedule, are all important factors. Even more so is the nature of the doctor–patient relationship, the degree to which a patient trusts his doctor, likes, admires and even loves him, or dislikes him. Some of the reactions of a patient depend on his intelligence and social sophistication, on his cultural background, how he looks on a drug and its likely effects. And even the most well informed of us still have a need for magic, are still, beneath our cultivated exteriors, irrational.

Today we are inundated with controlled trials of new drugs. Most of them contribute almost nothing to clinical understanding and wisdom. Indeed, since their results and conclusions are so often contradictory, the effect is confusing. The reason for this is that the patients making up most drug trials are clinically heterogenous; depression for instance is a protean term and there is no uniform agreement about terminology. Drugs are given for comparatively short periods, the dosage is often inadequate, and the results of such trials depend more on arbitrary rating scales than on clinical perceptiveness.

When a drug really works it is obvious to everyone, doctor and patient. That impramine and amitriptyline are most useful in endogenous types of depression, and the MAOIs particularly effective in reactive depression, became apparent to most clinical psychiatrists within 1 or 2 years of these drugs being introduced. It hardly required laborious double blind controlled trials to prove this point, any more than did streptomycin's efficacy in tuberculous meningitis.

Double blind trials in psychiatry are, on the whole, valueless; their instigators all too often pretend to be 'scientific', and rely on questionnaires rather than clinical ability. The essential requirements for useful research into psychotropic drugs are, understanding the natural history of the condition under investigation, the patience to undertake a painstaking selection of patients, and the ability to analyse the responses of patients to the treatment under study. In many instances, uncontrolled drug trials have yielded more information than double blind controlled studies.

Polypharmacy is, regrettably, often needed in psychiatry. Depression is frequently accompanied by anxiety or agitation of such intensity that an antidepressant drug alone is not enough; a tranquilliser must then be added. An anti-Parkinsonian drug may have to be given concomitantly with a neuroleptic to counteract its extrapyramidal effects. An antidepressant drug may have to be prescribed to a depressed schizophrenic receiving monthly injections of fluphenazine or flupenthixol.

Many drugs interact and have antagonistic, synergistic or additive effects, which can occasionally be fatal. One drug may prevent the absorption of another, compete for binding sites on plasma proteins or receptors, inhibit or stimulate catabolising enzymes, enhance or diminish renal clearance. It is essential to recognise such possible interactions before prescribing a second or third drug to a patient.

Pharmacokinetic studies are still young, but suggest that genetic factors are responsible for individual differences in the rate at which a drug is metabolised, and the extraordinary wide variation in effective drug dosage that exists. Depending on the drug, absorption occurs from the stomach, and later from the intestine. The degree and rapidity of absorption are affected by various factors: content of the gastric juice, motility, diet, and the presence of other drugs. Once absorbed, drugs pass to the liver and are metabolised, sometimes into therapeutically active metabolites; for instance amitriptyline to nortriptyline, diazepam to medazepam. From there the drug, its concentration by now reduced, passes to the brain. Giving a drug by injection allows it direct access to the brain, without alteration in the liver.

The activity of the microsomal enzymes of the liver, responsible for drug metabolism, is stimulated by some drugs, inhibited by others. The most important from a clinician's point of view are alcohol, barbiturates, phenytoin, and possibly phenothiazine derivatives. A heavy drinker who continues to drink may well need a bigger dose of an antidepressant drug than a nondrinker. So also may the patient who regularly takes a barbiturate at bedtime. A few drugs, notably the MAOIs and progesterone, inhibit liver enzymes and thereby lessen drug metabolism. A woman taking one of the progesterone-containing contraceptive pills may therefore need a smaller dose than otherwise of an antidepressant or tranquilliser; and if she stops the contraceptive pill, the dosage of the drug, to remain effective, may need to be increased. Needless to say, extreme caution is necessary if psychotropic drugs have to be given to anyone with serious liver damage.

In the blood stream most psychotropic drugs, with the exception of lithium, are bound to plasma proteins, in which form they are inactive. Only 10 to 20 per cent of a drug is free and therefore active. Measurement of the concentration of a drug is still largely a matter of research interest. However, it may well have a useful part to play in the future in the treatment of intractable depression.

Lithium exists free and active in the plasma, and it is important that its concentration in the blood should lie between 0·6 and 1·2 mmol/l for it to be effective in controlling most cases of manic depression.

Reports that antidepressant drugs, such as nortriptyline, are ineffective below 50 ng/ml are understandably consistent. But that levels above 250 ng/ml are also ineffective is difficult to accept, particularly when reports are contradictory Clinically there are patients who respond only when very large doses of an antidepressant drug are given. Of course such patients may absorb only part of the dosage, or the drug may be metabolised excessively rapidly, or virtually all of it be bound to plasma proteins. Much more work is needed on the subject before we can afford to be dogmatic about dosage. It is important for the clinican to recognise that each patient is unique, and has his own optimum drug dosage.

Excretion takes place largely through the kidneys. Renal damage or conditions such as cardiac failure which impair excretion invariably reduce the rate at which drugs are removed from the body. Apart from lithium, only a small proportion of any psychotropic drug is excreted unchanged in the urine; for instance, less than 30 per cent of imipramine. How often a drug needs to be given to maintain an effective concentration in the blood obviously depends largely on the speed at which it is metabolised, and if metabolites are active. Some drugs must be taken three or four times a day, for instance, nomifensine, others, like amitriptyline, once a day. And a drug such as penfluridol, which has an extremely slow rate of excretion, once a week.

Pharmacogenetics have proved of increasing if limited usefulness. A depressed patient with say a first-degree relative who responded to a particular antidepressant in the past, is more likely to be helped by that drug or its close analogue than one of a different class. Of course, to have had a close relative who responded well to drug which is then prescribed for oneself may well heighten its placebo effect. A genetic explanation is not necessarily the only one possible.

Lastly, it is always important to question the possible reasons for a patient not responding to drug treatment after reasonable length of time. Is the dosage too low? Is the patient really taking the drug regularly? Are the effects of the drug being countered by alcohol or another drug? Are unsuspected organic factors playing a part? Or is the diagnosis wrong? All these matters should be considered before new treatment is instigated.

PART 2. ANTIDEPRESSANTS

In the past depression was treated in a variety of ways, by isolation and rest, shocks, mesmerism and so on. Particularly when accompanied by much anxiety, opium or one or more of a large range of sedatives were employed; the most popular of which, just before the advent of the psychotropic drugs, were bromides and barbiturates. In the 1930s the amphetamines were introduced, and they and related compounds were virtually the only drugs available for the treatment of depression until 1957. But their euphoric effect was short-lived, and their disadvantages were considerable; their usefulness in fact, in the vast majority of depressed patients, was negligible. E.c.t., introduced in 1937, was the only treatment that truly relieved depression. But by no means all patients responded to e.c.t., or if they did they were liable to relapse within a few weeks; and side effects, particularly disturbance of memory, were sometimes upsetting.

In 1952 iproniazid was used in the treatment of tuberculosis and seen to have a remarkable if unexpected stimulating effect on patients. It was shown to be an inhibitor of MAO, but interest in the drug lapsed until the introduction of reserpine. Reserpine and chlorpromazine were given for the treatment of depression in the early 1950s, but results were not encouraging. However, interest in reserpine increased when it was discovered that it was itself liable to produce depression in about 15 per cent of patients treated with the drug, either for psychiatric purposes or hypertension. This depressant action was believed to be mediated through depletion of the storage and concentration of monoamines in the brain. New interest was now taken in iproniazid, which was indeed found to relieve some states of depression. It seemed possible that the anti-depressive effect of iproniazid was due to its ability to inhibit MAO, and so increase the concentration of monoamines in the brain. Confirmation followed when it was found that iproniazid could abolish the depressive syndrome produced by reserpine in laboratory animals.

Iproniazid began to be used clinically in 1957. Almost at once another compound, imipramine, was discovered, again by accident, to be an effective antidepressant. Its structure and properties were unlike those of iproniazid; it did not inhibit MAO. But like iproniazid it was capable of increasing the concentration of monoamines at receptor sites in the brain. It did this not by inhibiting MAO, but by blocking the reuptake of monoamines released in the synaptic cleft.

Suddenly then, in 1957, two potent antidepressant drugs became available to clinicians and an exciting field of research into the biochemical basis of depression appeared. Inevitably there was clinical confusion at first, and exaggerated claims for each drug or group of drugs were made. Gradually, with increasing experience, the picture has cleared, although by no means completely.

We know that the MAOIs are particularly useful in reactive types of depression and anxiety states, and that endogenous depression responds much better to imipramine and the other tricyclic analogues. However, not only is this classification still controversial, but it is admittedly often difficult to decide whether a depression is reactive or endogenous. All too often the clinical state is a mixed one, with reactive and endogenous features. The idea that a reactive depression always has clear cut external causes, while an endogenous depression has none, or insufficient to account for such depression, is of course misleading; a minority of patients conform to textbook stereotypes. For the most part, clinicians must depend on signs and symptoms, the length and course of the illness, the family history of affective disorder and its response to treatment, the patient's personality and life style. The need to make a diagnosis is no longer simply an academic exercise; the type of treatment prescribed, whether a MAOI, tricyclic, or other drug or combination of drugs, is dependent on this. It requires not only the most careful scrutiny of the patient and his symptoms, but also the use of that subtle intuitive sense which develops (and which is all too often suppressed today) with experience. To judge by the remarks of some practitioners, treating a depressed patient is a simple clockwork exercise; you prescribe the 'safest' and latest antidepressant and gradually work your way along the drug line, often bypassing the MAOIs because of their 'dangers', often using unsuitable dosages, until eventually e.c.t. is suggested as a last resort. This of course makes a mockery of psychiatry. We may still be a long way from becoming scientists, but we do have effective tools at our disposal now, and they demand expertise. Just as the poor workman blames his tools for bad work, so today the poor psychiatrist blames his failures on his drugs. Only by understanding to the full the effects of the antidepressant drugs now available, and the differing ways in which they interact with individual patients, and among themselves, can clinical psychiatrists expect their treatment to succeed.

Tricyclic antidepressants

The molecules of all these substances include three joined rings, differing from the phenothiazine nucleus in having seven atoms instead of six in the central ring (Fig. 1.1). It is this ring structure which gives the drug its antidepressant quality. Variations in the side chain attached to the central ring (R2), and in the atom at R1, account for differences in potency and sedative action between individual tricyclics. (Table. 1.1)

Imipramine and amitriptyline are the oldest and best established members of the tricyclic group. Today there are more than 12 potent derivatives of this molecular structure. Biochemically they vary. Some predominantly inhibit the reuptake of noradrenaline (NA)—for instance nortriptyline, desipramine, and the quadricyclic maprotiline. Others inhibit 5HT reuptake, especially clomipramine. Most of the others inhibit the reuptake of both 5HT and catecholamines in differing degrees. Some, such as trimipramine, appear not to influence the reuptake of either substance. This knowledge is not simply of academic interest, for it can sometimes be usefully applied clinically, albeit clumsily. Catecholamine reuptake inhibitors are best when reactive elements are prominent; 5HT reuptake inhibitors with biopolar depressions.

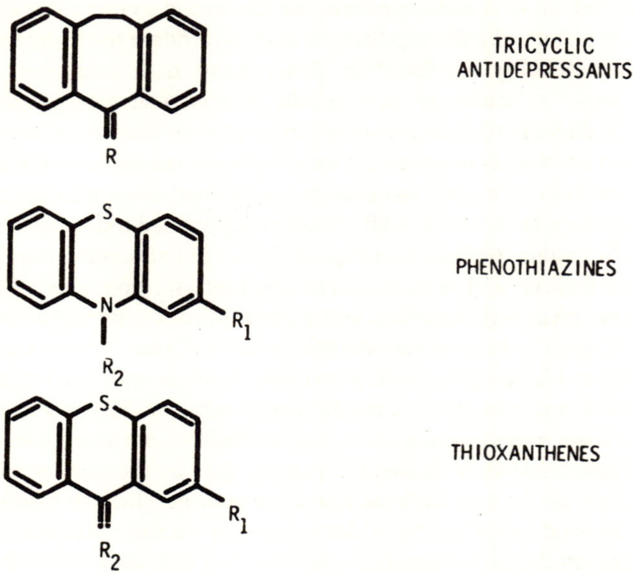

Fig. 1.1

Depression is protean, and it is easy for the unwary to overlook the possibility of depressive illness. Many patients present with anxiety and worry, especially about their health. Physical symptoms are common, abdominal pain, headache, back pain, and muscle discomfort. Unusual, irresponsible behaviour may mask depression.

The tricyclic antidepressants not only elevate mood, restore energy and

Table 1.1 Classification of thymoleptics (From Dally, P.J. 1978. Drug therapy. In *Therapy Options in Psychiatry*. Ed. Connolly, J. Pitman Medical)

1.	**Tricyclic antidepressants**	
	Amitriptyline	Butriptyline
	Imipramine	Desipramine
	Nortriptyline	Clomipramine
	Trimipramine	Protriptyline
2.	**Tricyclic-based compounds**	
	Dothiepin	Nomifensine
	Dibenzepin	Doxepin
3.	**Tetracyclic antidepressants**	
	Maprotiline	Mianserin
4.	**Oxazines**	
	Viloxazine	

drive, lift depression and lessen tension, they also sedate, in some cases excessively. Their usefulness, by and large, is in the treatment of endogenous states of depression; with broken sleep and early morning waking, lack of appetite, sometimes with severe weight loss, anergia, absent libido, self blame and guilt, depression at times serious enough for suicide to be contemplated, improving towards evening, and varying degrees of retardation and agitation. In the most severe cases psychotic symptoms develop.

The reactive depressions which respond so well to MAOIs are more akin to anxiety states; depression is not so deep, autonomic functions not so seriously upset, and the patient often angrily blames others for his misfortunes, seeing himself the victim rather than the cause of his troubles. Imipramine and amitryptyline have been consistently shown to be superior to MAOIs such as phenelzine and tranylcypromine, in endogenous depression. Seventy to 80 per cent of mildly depressed patients respond within a fortnight to amitriptyline; often with a comparatively small dose of around 75 mg at night. Even smaller doses are effective in the elderly. But when depression is severe the tricyclic antidepressants may not be adequate. Certainly, if suicide is a risk, then e.c.t. should never be delayed, particularly in view of the comparatively long interval between starting an antidepressant and its therapeutic effect.

However, a tricyclic can be safely combined with e.c.t., and by the time several e.c.t. have been given its antidepressant effects are emerging. Not only does this reduce the number of treatments needed, but the risk of subsequent relapse is greatly reduced.

There are clinicians who maintain that there is little to choose between the antidepressant effectiveness of the various tricyclics, and it is only the patient's intolerance to different side effects which makes one drug seem preferable or superior to another. The same used to be said of the neuroleptics. Certainly the unpleasantness of side effects may make it impossible to give an adequate dose. But there are good clinical reasons for thinking that clomipramine is better in depression associated with obsessional/compulsive symptoms, and in some cases of manic depression, while nortriptyline and the quadricyclic maprotiline often seem most effective when stressful reactive factors are prominent.

Of course the ability of a drug to sedate is also a reason why one tricyclic is preferred to another (Table. 1.2). Amitriptyline is more sedating than imipramine or clomipramine, and is the first choice when dealing with an agitated depression. Trimipramine is most sedating of all the tricyclics and is ideal for treating very tense anxious patients, constantly complaining of broken sleep and early morning anxiety. On the other hand, its antidepressant qualities are low and, on its own, it is no substitute for amitriptyline in serious depression.

Table 1.2 Alerting effects of thymoleptics (From Dally, P.J. 1978. Drug therapy. In *Therapy Options in Psychiatry*. Ed. Connolly, J. Pitman Medical)

Stimulating	Neutral	Sedating
Imipramine	Nortriptyline	Trimipramine
Desipramine	Dibenzepin	Amitriptyline
Protriptyline	Dothiepin	Doxepin
Nomifensine	Clomipramine	Mianserin
Viloxazine	Butriptyline	Maprotiline

Amitriptyline has been consistently shown to be better than or as good as any other tricyclic, and it is used in comparative trials of new antidepressants. Imipramine is as potent an antidepressant, but is less sedating; its use is particularly indicated in retarded depression, when a patient is slowed up physically and mentally, and perhaps is developing paranoid delusions.

Side effects of all the tricyclics vary enormously from one patient to another. These depend not only on dosage but also on individual susceptibility, influenced by age and sex, on a patient's tolerance, and his motivation and belief in the drug (and his doctor). There is nearly always some degree of placebo response, positive or negative, which for the most part tends to diminish and disappear over a few weeks. If severe unpleasant side effects continue, despite lowering the dose, there is little point in persisting with the drug.

Old people are particularly sensitive to anticholinergic side effects,and can develop alarming hypotension and states of confusion. Dothiepin and doxepin, which are very similar structurally, are less liable to cause such effects, particularly when small doses are given initially and only increased slowly. Doxepin and the quadricyclic mianserin are currently recommended for patients with heart disease, particularly ischaemic disease affecting the conduction bundles.

In severe depression tricyclic antidepressant effects may understandably take longer to manifest themselves. Certainly the maximum response may not be reached for 2 months. Most clinicians are not prepared to wait such a time, to allow their patients to continue suffering, particularly when there can be no sure guarantee that the drug will eventually triumph. After raising the dosage to as high a level as the patient can tolerate, if there is no obvious lift within a month it is better to change to another class of antidepressant, or consider e.c.t.

Occasionally the combination of two tricyclic antidepressants is effective when one is not. For instance, trimipramine at bedtime can be usefully combined with imipramine or amitriptyline during the daytime. Trimipramine is a splendid hypnotic and sedative, with none of the depressing effects that a diazepine, and even small doses of a neuroleptic sometimes have. A depressed patient, unable to sleep for long, agitated and restless, may improve quickly with 100 mg trimipramine and 100 mg or more of amitriptyline or clomipramine; side effects, apart from dryness of the mouth, are not prominent. If necessary, a hypnotic may also be given.

In the belief that 5HT is depleted in both mania and depression, and that NA is depleted in depression and raised in mania, a combination of clomipramine and maprotiline has been suggested for treating depressed manic depressives. Giving 50 to 100 mg of each drug together, we have not been impressed by the response of patients to date.

When a depressed patient is very agitated it is usually necessary to combine a tranquillising drug with the tricyclic. A small dose of a tranquilliser, a diazepine derivative or a neuroleptic, by quickly reducing tension, can sometimes lift mood on its own; but these drugs have no specific antidepressant properties. Severe tension and agitation are unpleasant for the patient and may well impede the action of the antidepressant. Comparatively large doses of diazepam, or one of its analogues, up to 80 mg a day, or chlorpromazine 150 to 300 mg a day, can be combined with an antidepressant without affecting the latter's activity. In fact there is evidence that phenothiazines may enhance the activity of tricyclic antidepressants by reducing their breakdown in the liver.

In therapeutically resistant cases of depression, when the response to tricyclics and MAOIs alone has been poor, the combination of a MAOI, preferably tranylcypromine, with a tricyclic, either trimipramine or amitriptyline, is sometimes most effective. The patient is typically a middle-aged perfectionist, has been increasingly tense for several years, and shows a mixture of reactive and endogenous depressive symptoms; early morning waking, with a heightened mood of despair, some but probably not marked loss of weight, a constant sense of anxiety and bodily tension, and a sense of inadequacy rather than guilt. Much has been written about the so-called dangers of this combination. But (provided the patient is reliable over his diet) the combination of a MAOI with such drugs as trimipramine, amitriptyline, imipramine and nortriptyline seems to be safe and effective. Only clomipramine with tranylcypromine, in our experience, has resulted in signs of cerebral overstimulation; sweating, pyrexia, twitching and disorientation. These disappeared within 12 hours of stopping all treatment. (Fuller details of combined antidepressant treatment are set out below, under the MAOIs.)

Other combinations of tricyclics with newer antidepressants, such as viloxazine, nomifensine and mianserin do not, as yet, appear to have any particular advantage. We have used maprotiline, up to 100 mg, with mianserin up to 60 mg a day, for comparatively mild depressive states over periods of up to 3 weeks. Much more work on these newer drugs is needed, particularly using large doses, identifying the type of depression each is most likely to relieve, before the effect of drug combinations can be properly assessed.

Tricyclics, like other antidepressant drugs, do not cure depressive illness, they relieve symptoms; in many instances they restore the patient to what feels to him to be normality. Most depressions remit spontaneously sooner or later, usually within 6 to 18 months, although occasionally they may rumble on for 2 or more years. If the antidepressant drug is stopped before spontaneous recovery, depressive symptoms recur, usually within a fortnight of withdrawing the drug. Resuming the drug usually, although not invariably, restores the situation. It is always best to reduce the dosage of the antidepressant slowly, over the course of 4 weeks, rather than stop it abruptly. Not only does this avoid possible withdrawal effects if the drug has been taken for some time, but warning signs that depression is beginning to return are quickly noticed, and the original dosage at once restored before depression can regain a foothold.

Chronic depressive states develop mainly in older patients. In such cases, or when depression drags on because of adverse unchangeable circumstances, an effective antidepressant drug must be continued for years. Treatment is also prolonged, even indefinitely, when depression recurs frequently, every year or more often. A small dose of the appropriate tricyclic is continued after recovery, say 50 mg of amitriptyline — the exact dosage is found by trial and error — combined where appropriate with lithium carbonate. If and when depression begins to make itself felt again the dosage is immediately increased. Alternatively those patients who know from experience that depression is likely to recur in the spring or autumn can increase the antidepressant a few weeks before the expected attack. Such depressions often run like clockwork, and the drug can be quickly reduced at the anticipated time of recovery.

Some of the most striking successes are on masked depressions. Adominal pain, facial pain, headache, discomfort behind the eyes, aching muscles, respond dramatically to antidepressant drugs when such symptoms are secondary to depression. It is of course essential to establish whether depression preceded the onset of such physical symptoms, or developed as an understandable reaction to physical pain and discomfort. Many of the first group of patients deny that they are depressed in mood, but readily admit to feeling tired and irritable, lacking zest, being intolerant of noise, and to sleeping badly for some time prior to the onset of pain. Abdominal pain is a common symptom of depression. In many cases symptoms respond best to maprotiline, or an MAOI, especially when the patient expresses strong feelings of resentment.

Antidepressant drugs, by improving mood, can often help a patient with a chronically painful disorder, for instance osteoarthritis, to tolerate his discomfort; depression is a secondary feature of the condition, but all too readily increases a patient's misery and incapacity.

Dosage and length of treatment

Many patients are inadequately treated with antidepressants. Of 100 patients referred to our outpatient clinic for depression, the majority had already been prescribed an antidepressant, well below the therapeutic dose. Of course, there are wide individual differences due to different rates of absorption, metabolism and excretion, which we have already discussed. A maximum therapeutic range is claimed to exist, levels above which lessen the therapeutic response. This claim has been disputed. And certainly in practice the dosage of any antidepressant is more often than not determined by the side effects it causes, and the patient's ability to tolerate these.

But frequently a patient fails to respond to a particular drug because it has not been given in adequate dosage. Another common mistake is to start treatment with too large a dose of the tricyclic, with the result that the patient is so upset by side effects that he refuses to continue with that drug.

Unless a patient is so ill that he needs to be heavily sedated and confined to bed, or is impatient for results and is prepared to accept unpleasant side effects, it is best to start with a comparatively small dose and work slowly up to the maximum the patient can tolerate. For instance, a patient begins with 50 mg of amitriptyline at bedtime, doubles this after 3 days, and increases to 150 mg at the end of a week. By the end of the second week it should be apparent whether or not the drug is likely to be effective, even though maximal improvement may take up to 8 weeks. If after 2 weeks there is little sign of depressive symptoms lifting, and side effects are negligable, the dosage should be increased over the course of a further week to 300 mg; the maximum dosage of amitriptyline we have given has been 600 mg. When a patient responds to so high a dose it is sensible, after a few weeks, to attempt to reduce it to a lower level. On very high doses patients tend to be unstable in mood, liable at times to swing into hypomania, and may in consequence be difficult to manage.

With older patients in particular a comparatively small dose, 75 mg or even 50 mg of amitriptyline or dothiepin (better for old patients because of its lesser anticholinergic effects) is sufficient, and safer. We have had patients with long-standing anxiety-depressive states, who have never been able to tolerate more than 50 mg of amitriptyline, respond to this dosage over the course of 2 to 3 months, and are ultimately maintained on 10 to 20 mg at night. We do not believe that these are placebo responders.

Tricyclics, like other antidepressants, suppress symptoms; they do not cure depression. Since the vast majority of depressives cure themselves eventually it is necessary for the antidepressant to be continued, in the smallest effective dosage, until this time. A tricyclic therefore may need to be continued for months or years, or can be stopped after a few weeks. The problem clearly is to know when to stop. Some patients with recurring disorders are always depressed for the same period of time. Some patients are able to recognise when their (usually recurrent) depression has lifted and have no qualms or difficulty over stopping. Others, who may have been maintained on the drug for a year or more, are hesitant and reluctant to discard what they have come to regard as their life line. In any case, if a patient has been on a tricyclic for 6 months or more it is necessary to stop the drug slowly to avoid withdrawal effects. Suddenly stopping 100 mg trimipramine, after 2 years, resulted in nightmares and anxiety symptoms which ceased immediately trimipramine was resumed; 6 weeks were needed before the drug could be completely withdrawn without adverse effects. The simplest method of determining if a patient on, say amitriptyline 100 mg, is ready to stop the drug, is to reduce the dosage by 25 mg a week. If at any point symptoms of depression begin to return, the dosage must be restored and the procedure repeated in 3 months' time.

Overdosage

Anything above 10 times the therapeutic dose of any tricyclic is liable to be lethal. Overdosage results in delirium, convulsions, hyperpyrexia, hyperreflexia, bowel and bladder paralysis, and mydriasis. Tachycardia and arrhythmias can progress to cardiac arrest and death. Coma rarely lasts longer than 24 hours. The most important aspect of treatment is management of cardiac function, and ideally the patient should be admitted as soon as possible to an intensive care unit. Cardiac irregularities can develop several days after a patient has regained consciousness.

Side effects

Most side effects develop immediately. Although related to dosage, there are wide differences among patients. It is striking that patients with endogenous depressions usually experience less troublesome effects than those with reactive depression; MAOI responders in particular are liable to react very badly to tricyclics. Drowsiness is common at the start of treatment but lessens after 3 or 4 days, and often disappears as the drug's therapeutic effects appear. It can occur with all the tricyclics, but is likely to be greater with trimipramine and amitriptyline. A dry mouth is most unpleasant, and there is little to be done about it, apart from sucking fruit drops. Sweating over the upper half of the body is most common with imipramine. Constipation may need to be countered by laxatives; occasionally a patient develops loose motions. Urinary retention can be troublesome, especially in the elderly and those with prostatic enlargement. Sexual libido is sometimes reduced or lost, orgasm delayed or lost in either sex, and erection difficult. Vision is sometimes blurred due to difficulty in focussing. Narrow angle glaucoma can be made worse; but many patients with glaucoma can be successfully treated with tricyclics, although it is wise for an opthalmologist to give his approval. Gastro-intestinal functions are affected in several ways; the oesophageal sphincter relaxes, which may cause a patient with hiatus hernia to complain of increased discomfort, there is reduced gastric free acid secretion, and gastric motility diminishes; this can benefit patients with an irritable bowel syndrome. Rarely paralytic ileus develops, usually with large doses and after several weeks; the tricyclic must be stopped at once, although it can be resumed in a lower dosage when bowel movements have recovered. Tremor of limbs may affect handwriting, and can sometimes be so extreme as to require the drug to be stopped. Craving for carbohydrates often develops and may cause large weight gains.

Postural hypotension is particularly hazardous in elderly patients; drugs such as methylphenidate and dihydroergotamine do not provide a satisfactory answer, and the dosage must usually be reduced if falls are likely. Tachycardia is usual. In therapeutic doses tricyclics can cause e.c.g. changes; flattened T waves, prolonged Q T intervals, depressed S T segments. Because of their anticholinergic effects and the increased tissue level of catecholamines, all the tricyclics are probably capable of interfering with intracardiac conduction, especially in overdosage, or when the heart is already diseased; occasionally they lead to cardiac arrest and death. Doxepin appears to be safest in this respect. Congestive heart failure may be precipitated or worsened if present, and is a contraindication to using tricyclics.

C.n.s. effects are unusual. Epilepsy occasionally develops — maprotiline seems to be one of the worst offenders. But tricyclics do not seem to disturb the balance of an epileptic well controlled by anti-epileptic drugs. Treated epilepsy is not a contraindication to treatment with a tricyclic. (However, it should be remembered that phenytoin increases the rate of catabolism of tricyclics in the liver.) Parkinsonism and other extrapyramidal syndromes are rare occurences; since tricyclics possess strong anticholinergic actions, there is no point in prescribing orphenadrine.

Hypomania can be precipitated, schizophrenic features may develop, and psychopathic behaviour be released, usually as a result of high dosage and/or clinical oversight. Confusional states are particularly likely to develop in elderly patients, or when brain function is already impaired, as in incipient delirium tremens. Sleep is usually improved, but may be upset, especially by the less sedating antidepressants. Vivid dreams and nightmares can be particularly troublesome.

Which tricyclics to use and when?

There are now at least 12 tricyclic antidepressants available. It is only necessary to use four or five of them, but it is essential that the clinician knows each of these throughly.

Amitriptyline is the first choice in agitated depression, but in older patients *dothiepin*, although not as potent an antidepressant, is preferable, being less likely to cause confusion and troublesome anticholinergic side effects. *Imipramine* is indicated in retarded depression. It is liable initially to increase agitation, and if this is present to any marked degree imipramine should be combined with a tranquillising drug. *Clomipramine* is prescribed for the depressive phase of manic depression. Clomipramine is also useful for obsessional/compulsive and phobic anxiety states which are secondary to depressive illness.

Rapid therapeutic effects may be produced by intravenous infusion of clomipramine in normal saline. It is advisable, before starting such treatment to make sure the e.c.g. is normal. After a test dose of 25 mg, to identify idiosyncratic reactions the dosage is raised by 50 mg a day to the maximum of tolerance, which may be as high as 800 mg; the drug is given over 2 to 3 hours. Pulse and blood pressure should be recorded every 15 minutes. The dosage is then reduced by 75 mg a day and oral clomipramine substituted; the oral daily dosage is between 75 to 150 mg. The placebo effect is considerable and may go some way to account for the greater effectiveness of clomipramine given by infusion compared to the oral route. The main side effects of clomipramine infusion are sleepiness, hypotension—and occasionally hypertension—tachycardia, tremor, difficulty in micturition,haemolysis and haematuria rarely, and fits.

Trimipramine is most appropriate when a patient is very anxious, and waking after 2 or 3 hours in a state of tension. It is the most sedating of all the tricyclics and, for outpatients, is best reserved for night time. It does not suppress REM sleep. It can be combined with any other tricyclic, and with a MAOI. It is liable to cause confusion and unpleasant dreams in old age, and some alcoholic patients.

Maprotiline, which specifically blocks reuptake of catecholamines, is especially useful in mixed types of depression, where reactive factors and anxiety are prominent, tension has been high for some years, and insomnia, both initial and early wakening, is troublesome, but weight loss and the depth of depression are not severe. This is the type patient who has not done well with other tricyclics, and who might seem most suitable for treatment with combined antidepressants.

It is important to remember that when a patient has been successfully treated in the past with a particular antidepressant, or when a close relative of the patient has suffered from depression and responded to a specific drug, that antidepressant is the natural first choice.

Contraindications

1. Confusional states
2. Recent myocardial damage, particularly if this involves the conduction system
3. Cardiac failure
4. Caution is needed with glaucoma, prostatic enlargement, old age, liver failure.

Pregnancy

Ideally no woman should be on drugs if she is likely to become pregnant. But a patient may be on a tricyclic when she inadvertently conceives. There is no evidence that any of tricyclics causes damage to the foetus. Many patients have been treated throughout pregnancy with antidepressants, with no ill effects to themselves or the foetus. But obviously it is better to reduce and stop the drug if this is possible, provided alarm is not raised in the woman. Tricyclics enter breast milk, but in small amounts, and there is no reason on this account to prevent a mother who wishes to breastfeed from doing so.

New tricyclic-like compounds

Maprotiline is structurally like the tricyclics, with a fourth ring lying in the middle perpendicular to the others. It is therefore labelled quadricyclic. It is similar to the tricyclics in its metabolism. Biochemically it specifically blocks the reuptake of catecholamines, and barely affects 5HT. It does not suppress REM sleep. It has a long half-life, about 50 hours, and therefore can be given in a single dose at bedtime. Side effects increase with dosage. Anticholinergic effects are less, dose for dose, than say with amitriptyline. Skin rashes occur in about 10 per cent of patients, fits in about 1 per cent and cardiotoxicity is similar to the tricyclics. The dosage is 25 to 200 mg a day, most patients needing 75 to 100 mg. Overdose is similar in its effects to that of tricyclics.

It is particularly effective in anxiety-depression, in the presence of strong reactive factors, and tension which has been increasing for a year or more. Patients who respond are likely to have that mixture of obsessionality and immaturity in their make up which so often characterises the MAOI responder. These patients sometimes do badly with other tricyclic compounds, and respond only partially to combined antidepressants. Maprotiline does not seem to be helpful in serious endogenous depressive states. Indeed, in some cases of manic depression, it appears to increase agitation.

Mianserin. Although like maprotiline, it is a quadricyclic compound, *mianserin* has a different structure and different biochemical activities. It does not affect 5HT and NA reuptake. It has been suggested that its biochemical action is on presynaptic receptors, which control the release of monoamines in the synapse. As a serotonin antagonist it may produce a relative NA excess.

Mianserin has a short half-life and needs to be given at least twice and possibly three times a day to maintain adequate plasma levels. Side effects are few, mainly drowsiness. It has little anticholinergic activity, its cardiotoxicity is low, and it does not cause fits. Overdose does not therefore have the same dangers as with the tricyclics or maprotiline, and no deaths have been reported so far.

The drug has been compared favourably with amitriptyline, but none of the trials so far is impressive or of much clinical help. The type of patient most likely to respond to mianserin has still to be defined; but its action in severe depression seems to be negligible. The dosage varies between 30 and 300 mg a day in three divided doses.

L-tryphtophan is a precursor of the neurotransmitter 5HT. If depression is a result of lowered levels of 5HT, giving 5-hydroxytryptophan should bring about improvement. In fact, reports on the effectiveness of this substance in depression have not been encouraging. For the most part L-tryptophan seems to have little effect in depression of any severity, reactive or endogenous. Unlike some researchers, we have not found that it potentiates the MAOIs. On the other hand it does sometimes enhance the effect of clomipramine, a selective blocker of 5HT reuptake.

L-hydroxytryphtophan is sometimes useful in the treatment of depressed old people. Such patients may respond well to a dosage of between 1·5 and 7·0 g a day, even when agitated. There are no side effects apart from sleepiness and occasional gastro-intestinal discomfort.

Thyrotropic hormone and liothyronine. Thyrotropic hormone has not fulfilled earlier claims of effectiveness in depression.

Small doses of liothyronine (T3) are said to enhance the action of tricyclic antidepressants. Some reactively depressed middle-aged females do appear to helped by this combination; the dosage lies between 40 and 80 μg a day. It may be that T3 sensitises receptors and allows the tricyclic drug to exert a greater effect.

Monoamine oxidase inhibitors (MAOI)

The MAOIs have a much narrower range of usefulness than the tricyclics. Nonetheless, their action is often specific and unique, and patients crippled by their symptoms for years, who have failed to respond to a multitude of treatments, suddenly and dramatically begin to return to normal when given a MAOI. Much nonsense about the dangers of the MAOIs is promulgated; patients are often denied their benefit for this reason and allowed to drift, with their families, into a state of hopelessness and chronicity. It is surely time that all clinicians recognised the great value as well as the limitations of the MAOI.

For practical purposes there are four MAOIs—iproniazid, phenelzine, isocarboxazid and tranylcypromine. Although overlapping, each drug differs subtly in its effects from its companions, and therefore on the type of patient most likely to respond.

Phenelzine is a hydrazine derivative which has been in clinical use for over 20 years. It became clear, after using phenelzine and iproniazid on a wide range of patients, that these drugs were most useful in reactive or, what we called 'atypical or hysterical depression'. In these conditions anxiety is the predominant feature, and depression sometimes seems to be of secondary importance. Indeed, some people say that phenelzine should not be called an antidepressant, and that its central action is anxiolytic. These atypical depressions were often the most difficult to treat in the past. Psychotherapy frequently seemed to have no effect; electroshock often did more harm than good; and sedatives and tranquillisers given to relieve tension left the patient feeling more depressed and slowed down.

Symptoms vary widely in content and severity. The patient may complain of a constant yet irrational dread of impending disaster, or somatic symptoms such as headache, palpitations and muscular pains come to dominate his life and his mind. Sometimes anxiety becomes attached to outside objects and situations; phobias of harming people, travelling, or going out alone are common, and the picture is often similar to that of anxiety hysteria. Occasionally frank hysterical conversions occur, and we have seen fugues and amnesic states which did not clear up fully until the underlying depression was recognised and treated with phenelzine.

Clinically these patients show few signs of endogenous depression. They tend to project rather than introject their feelings, and blame other people rather than themselves for their plight. Sleep disturbance takes the form more of difficulty in getting to sleep than early morning waking; in fact these patients may be sleeping heavily when it is time to get up and have the utmost difficulty in waking. Instead of feeling worse in the first half of the day and then steadily improving, they are at their best early on and feel dreadful later in the day. An almost constant feature in women is marked exacerbation of symptoms a week or 10 days before their periods.

Sometimes symptoms have been present for years, or have run a chronic phasic course, and the patient has come to be looked upon by his relatives and doctor as a difficult neurotic for whom little can be done. In other cases symptoms develop rapidly after some special, often prolonged, stress. For instance, a middle-aged woman devotedly cared for her bed-ridden mother for 2 years, and at the same time held a responsible job. A month after her mother's death, she developed an overwhelming fear of going out alone. She had to give up her job and over the next 6 months became a miserable recluse. Another woman, with an unsatisfactory marriage, drifted into an affair with one of her husband's employees. Feelings of guilt were suppressed, but somatic symptoms became increasingly prominent and continued long after the affair had ended. Both these women recovered only when treated with phenelzine and chlordiazepoxide.

Although these patients may be regarded as neurotic or inadequate personalities, this is not really so. One of the characteristics of exogenous depressions responding to phenelzine is that the patients are well able to cope with their problems before they break down. Typically they tend to be obsessional, sensitive, highly strung people, with energy, drive and imagination. Beneath a confident exterior is an insecure, emotionally immature person, dependent upon success and approval to maintain psychic defences. Often they have overreactive autonomic systems, which accounts for some of their symptoms. Frequently they push themselves to the limit of their capacity, and in spite of disabling symptoms try to carry on with their work.

People with lifelong inadequate personalities may present with rather similar symptoms, but they are not helped by phenelzine. In fact, such patients may become more tense, and in some cases inhibitions are lessened, releasing irresponsible and antisocial behaviour. Generally they respond better to tranquillisers or flupenthixol. Before these were available they were helped by barbiturates; but there is a serious risk of addiction in this type of patient. This emphasises the importance of understanding the premorbid personality; and that of course requires a full and perceptive history. Psychiatrists who take no trouble with their histories cannot expect to distinguish the advantage of one drug over another, and they can anticipate making the same mistake over and over again. Phenelzine will not help a patient who, since childhood, has constantly proved unable to cope with relatively minor difficulties.

Where anxiety is very marked, the effect of phenelzine is enhanced by combining it with a tranquillising drug. Phobic anxiety and somatic anxiety symptoms, particularly tachycardia and palpitations, respond well to a combination of phenelzine and chlordiazepoxide, while free floating anxiety is better treated by combining phenelzine with one of piperazine phenothiazines such as trifluoperazine (1 mg). Neither a tranquilliser nor phenelzine given alone is nearly as effective as the combination.

Patients with cardiac neurosis or effort syndrome, who rarely respond to simple reassurance, do particularly well with this combination of drugs. Palpitation, hyperventilation and pain over the heart may convince the patient that he has heart disease and lead to a vicious spiral of mounting anxiety and autonomic overactivity. Even when true angina is present, anxiety may increase symptoms out of all proportion. Treatment with phenelzine combined with chlordiazepoxide usually leads to marked improvement within 10 days. Fatigue is a common complaint of these patients, and many say that they wake up in the morning just as tired as when they went to bed. They feel drained of energy, dull and lacking all interest, and the smallest molehill becomes a mountain. Unlike a patient with endogenous depression, appetite for food and sex are often unaffected. They may sleep heavily both day and night. They look well. Small wonder that they receive scant sympathy and understanding from others.

Some psychosomatic symptoms also respond well to phenelzine (and tranylcypromine). Atypical facial pain, which on superficial examination may resemble trigeminal neuralgia, can totally disappear.

A woman of 42 gave an 8 year history of continuous pain over the left lower half of her face, and of increasing depression. She was an overconscientious woman, with acquaintances but no close friends; her sense of security and interests were centred on her family. For many years she had felt resentful towards her husband over his preference for night work. Eventually he gave into his wife's complaints and changed to day work. Almost immediately his firm ran into economic difficulties and he was made redundant. Six months later his wife developed pain in her face. Treatment ranged from the orthodox to esoteric, and included the loss of three healthy teeth, but without avail. She gave up her job, withdrew from social activities and became a miserable burden to herself and her family. On a combination of 45 mg phenelzine and 2 mg trifluoperazine a day her mood lifted and pain began to fade; after 8 weeks she was virtually pain-free. Three years later she still requires this combination; pain returns within a week of reducing the dosage.

In assessing such cases for treatment with phenelzine, it is important to obtain a history of emotional disturbances and anxiety and depression preceding the onset of pain. When depression follows pain, treatment may improve matters by lifting mood and so raising the patient's tolerance, but will not remove the pain.

Symptoms from an irritable bowel syndrome—abdominal pain alternating with constipation and diarrhoea—may also respond well to small doses of tricyclic antidepressants. Frequent loose bowel motions and frequency of urine all too readily become associated with phobic anxiety. In extreme cases this can result in a patient becoming virtually house-bound and unable to work. Phenelzine, with a tranquilliser, can reduce anxiety and autonomic activity sufficiently to allow the patient to deal with the problem and resume his normal life (see Ch. 5 Behavioural psychotherapy).

The usual effective daily dosage of phenelzine is 45 mg, but there is considerable individual variation. For outpatients it is advisable to start with 45 mg a day in three divided doses, and to warn the patient of possible side effects, and the need to avoid certain foods. If after a fortnight there is no improvement, and no troublesome side effects, the dosage should be raised to 60 mg a day (in three divided doses) then slowly to 90 mg a day, but few people can tolerate such a large dose for long.

Like the tricyclics there is a lag before improvement appears, but in the main, anxiety lessens and mood improves within a week. However, a fortnight should be allowed before increasing the dosage and assessing the outcome. Once it is clear that the patient is improving the dosage should be continued without change, unless side effects are a nuisance, for at least 6 weeks. Much depends on the patient's length of history and his circumstances, as to how long treatment with phenelzine needs to continue. As long as outside stresses remain and continue to feed the patient's tension, phenelzine usually has to be continued; the drug merely suppresses symptoms, which are liable to return within a week of stopping. Clearly, every effort must be made to help the patient solve his problems once he is feeling better, otherwise treatment will be prolonged. On the other hand, stresses which originally set the disorders going may have disappeared by the time the patient comes for treatment. Now anxiety and depression are kept going through a vicious circle effect, of habit and constitutional neurotic factors. Once phenelzine has broken the vicious circle, and helped to restore the patient's self-confidence, the dosage can be slowly reduced and treatment finished. Particularly if the drug has been taken for some months it should be stopped gradually; withdrawal effects, which include anxiety and the reactivation of symptoms, are otherwise likely.

Tranylcypromine is also a MAOI, but is not a hydrazine derivative. It has more distinctly antidepressant power than phenelzine. While phenelzine is indicated in long standing severe tension states, tranylcypromine is particularly valuable in reactive types of depression. When, as so often happens, the picture is mixed one, with endogenous features such as early morning waking, tranylcypromine combined with trimipramine is effective when all other treatments may have failed.

Tranylcypromine has similarities, both in structure and action to amphetamine. It can sometimes produce a sharp euphoric action within 48 to 72 hours, which later fades into the more steady antidepressant effect associated with MAOIs, which develops about a week after starting treatment. Patients with tension states may be upset by this stimulating effect, and their symptoms increased.

Tranylcypromine is particularly useful when somnolence and lethargy are prominent; these are present in some atypical depressive states. The patient complains that he is exhausted by the smallest exertion, mentally and physically, and he is liable to fall asleep if left undisturbed; he may spend 14 hours or more a day asleep, and the picture resembles narcolepsy. Amphetamine often helped this patient in the past, but its effect is erratic and tolerance all too often develops. Phenelzine may fail, but tranylcypromine can lift all these symptoms within a fortnight. Tranylcypromine is also useful in relieving the anergia of schizophrenia, particularly those whose psychoses have 'burnt out'. Tranylcypromine is not as effective as tricyclics in clear cut endogenous depression. In such cases the drug should be reserved for patients who have failed to respond to adequate treatment with tricyclics, and particularly when they are intolerant of their side effects, so that a high dosage is difficult to achieve.

Tranylcypromine can be usefully combined with other drugs. Anxiety and tension symptoms are common components of depression, and tranylcypromine alone may increase these, at least initially. A small dose of a piperazine phenothiazine, trifluoperazine 1 mg two or three times a day for instance, relieves tension without causing the sleepiness or dullness that sometimes follow diazepam.

The combination of tranylcypromine with a tricyclic antidepressant can succeed when all other treatments have failed, including e.c.t. The patient most likely to respond has been increasingly tense and depressed for some years. Physical symptoms like headache, nausea, and back pain are prominent. Phobic anxiety has reduced the patient's activities, concentration has declined and sleep is disturbed; the patient perhaps getting off but always waking in the early hours. The addition of trimipramine not only potentiates the antidepressant activity of tranylcypromine but also counteracts insomnia. The combination is a safe one, although hypotensive effects can be troublesome and restrict dosage. Other tricyclics and maprotiline may also be safely combined with tranylcypromine, particularly those which mainly inhibit the reuptake of NA; when early morning wakening is absent, amitriptyline or nortriptyline are more effective than trimipramine. Drugs such as clomipramine which inhibit 5HT reuptake, are most likely to cause dangerous cerebral effects. Some authorities suggest that the MAOI should be prescribed first, and the tricyclic added a week later. We find no advantage in this, and start combined treatment with both drugs simultaneously.

Some patients with recurrent depression, both bipolar and unipolar types, are helped actively and prophylactically by combining tranylcypromine with lithium carbonate. There are no additional problems with such a combination.

Side effects of MAOIs are few. Postural hypotension calls for a reduction of dosage when severe. Constipation is rarely troublesome. Ankle and periorbital oedema are sometimes sufficiently marked to require a diuretic. Insomnia is most likely with tranylcypromine. Twitching and explosive jerkings at night are worse with iproniazid; but may be relieved by diazepam or pyridoxine. Very rarely jaundice is caused by the hydrazine MAOIs, iproniazid more so than phenelzine; not by tranylcypromine. Headaches are most common with tranylcypromine, occuring in around 2 per cent of patients. As with all antidepressants, psychotic episodes can be precipitated.

Toxic effects are almost invariably the result of a patient eating forbidden foods, or taking proprietary cough and cold cures containing ephedrine or phenylpropanolamine. This can result in a hypertensive crisis and/or cerebral excitation; confusion, hyperpyrexia and convulsions.

A hypertensive crisis is due to the release of free catecholamines from binding sites. Pressor amines like tyramine, which is present in foods such as cheese, are normally broken down by MAOI in the gut wall and liver; but because MAO is inhibited they now pass directly into the circulation. Foods to avoid include cheese (except cottage cheese), yoghurt, yeast and meat extracts, pickled herring, paté, game, chianti wine, broad bean pods and banana skins. A severe, pounding, usually occipital headache develops, sometimes without warning, but often preceded by palpitations, with nausea and vomiting. Death can result from a hypertensive crisis, usually from rupture of an aneurysm on one of the cerebral vessels. Treatment is with 5 mg phentolamine i.v. if this is to hand; otherwise it is best to treat the patient conservatively, lying down and sedated with chlorpromazine or diazepam. The severe headache usually lifts within an hour, although an unpleasant dull headache may persist for some days afterwards.

Dangerous reactions can sometimes develop when drugs acting on the sympathetic nervous system are taken concurrently. Although amphetamine itself is compatible with the MAOI, ephedrine, phenylephrine and phenylpropanolamine can cause a hypertensive crisis. Dangerous reactions can also occur with methyldopa, L-dopa and clonidine. Narcotic analgesics like pethidine, morphine, cocaine and procaine may interact dangerously. Most anaesthetists, before cold surgery, require a

MAO inhibitor to be stopped a fortnight or so beforehand in case measures to restore blood pressure are required at operation. No tricyclic must be given parenterally until at least 14 days have elapsed after stopping the MAO inhibitor. The actions of barbiturates and alcohol are potentiated, and the effects of insulin and hypoglycaemic drugs increased by MAO inhibitors.

Dependence occurs virtually only with tranylcypromine, and always in patients with inadequate personalities who come to rely on the amphetamine-like effects. One of our patients was taking up to 400 mg a day.

The daily dose of phenelzine ranges from 30 to 90 mg, the usual being 45 mg a day, and of isocarboxazid from 20 to 60 mg. The daily dose of tranylcypromine is usually 20 to 40 mg, but can go up to 80 mg a day.

Contraindications to the MAO inhibitors

1. Severe cirrhosis or liver failure
2. Concurrently with certain drugs (see above)
3. A past history of subarachnoid haemorrhage
4. Prostatic enlargement sufficient to cause retention.

Lithium carbonate

Lithium is widely used to treat mania and to prevent recurrent affective disorders. Its mode of action is still speculative. It affects cell membranes; and may prevent the redistribution of intracellular sodium which occurs in many affective disorders. It influences neurotransmitters; increases the breakdown of catecholamines at presynaptic sites, blocks their release at synapses, and reduces the sensitivity of postsynaptic receptors. It may alter output of corticosteroids, which in turn affects the concentration and distribution of sodium and potassium. Lithium is readily absorbed, and is distributed evenly throughout the body. It can replace both sodium, which is mostly extracellular, and potassium which is mainly intracellular. It enters cells slowly, and its slowish rate of therapeutic action is probably dependent on this.

Cade in Australia reported on the efficacy of lithium salts in the treatment of psychotic excitement in 1949. Subsequently he used lithium to treat acute mania. The dosage needed is between 1000 and 2000 mg a day, which is approaching toxic levels. Weekly serum lithium levels are advisable in such circumstances, and a close watch kept for signs of toxicity. Lithium has the additional disadvantage in mania of requiring at least 10 days to take effect. Today there are more rapid and efficient methods of treating acute mania, using chlorpromazine and haloperidol, although lithium carbonate is often given concurrently.

Lithium carbonate is valuable in lessening or preventing recurrent affective disorders. The drug's prophylactic value in manic depression, or bipolar affective disorders is quite clear Lithium can sometimes abolish attacks completely. More commonly, the frequency of attacks is lessened and the severity of symptoms and their duration considerably diminished. Studies have shown that about 30 per cent of manic depressives on lithium relapse over a 2 year period, compared to 90 per cent on placebo. A small proportion of patients are not helped, and may even become more depressed during a depressive phase. There is no sure way of knowing in advance whether a patient will or will not respond to lithium. Only rapid cycling (four or more episodes over a year) is definitely associated with a poor response.

Most authorities agree that the unipolar affective disorders, or recurrent depression, also respond to lithium, although probably not so well as manic depression does. Conflicting reports may be due to the difficulty of being sure whether recurring depression is really unipolar or bipolar; and if unipolar, whether endogenous, reactive, or neurotic.

There is disagreement about the antidepressant activity of lithium. Some reports suggest that lithium is more effective than imipramine in bipolar depressive disorders, and equally effective in unipolar. Most clinicians agree that a depressed patient is better treated with antidepressant drugs, or e.c.t., than with lithium alone. However, many combine lithium with an antidepressant when treating recurrent depression. There is evidence that this combination may be more effective than either drug alone.

Schizophrenia is not helped by lithium prescribed on its own. But some schizo-affective disorders, with a strong affective component, undoubtedly do better when a neuroleptic is combined with lithium. Of course, some of these successes may conceivably be because manic depression has been mistaken for schizo-affective disorders. But there is growing evidence that lithium plus phenothiazine are better than a phenothiazine alone in schizophrenia accompanied by much depression.

Lithium has been reported to be useful in a variety of other disorders involving periodicity and disturbance of mood; premenstrual tension, alcoholism associated with depression, and aggressive psychopathic outbursts. However lithium is unlikely to be consistently useful in these conditions.

Long-term lithium should not be prescribed without good reason. Three episodes of manic depression involving at least one attack of mania, within 2 years, or an attack of depression each year for 3 or 4 years, unresponsive to maintenance treatment with antidepressants, are good reasons for considering lithium. Once begun, lithium may have to be given indefinitely. Even after 10 years of freedom from attack a patient developed mania 4 months after stopping lithium. Mild swings of depression and hypomania often occur during maintenance treatment, and may call for a temporary increase of lithium and/or the addition of haloperidol or an antidepressant.

Occasionally, having been effective for years, lithium ceases to protect. Mrs S. had her first attack of depression at 19, and of mania followed by depression at 26, after the birth of her only child. She was then free of symptoms until the age of 45. Attacks of alternating mania and depression then developed and recurred every 2 years in the spring, shortening to yearly intervals 12 years later. She started lithium at this time, and although not completely controlled, the severity of symptoms was considerably lessened. Oedema suddenly developed after 9 years, due apparently to the lithium, and coincidentally attacks of mania and depression increased in severity and periodicity. Over the past 3 years she has required large doses of neuroleptics, antidepressants and e.c.t. at different times, in spite of lithium levels remaining well within the therapeutic range.

The dosage of lithium, in the form of lithium carbonate, ranges from 400 to 1600 mg a day, most or all of which can be given once a day, preferably at bedtime. The aim is to achieve a steady serum concentration of between 0·8 and 1·2 mmol/l. However, it is a mistake to insist too rigidly on achieving these levels. Some manic depressive patients remain well and feel better on levels as low as 0·4 mmol/l. Careful observation and monitoring of the serum lithium concentration are needed for the first few weeks, but these can be gradually extended to 3 and then 6 monthly intervals, provided the patient and, just as important, her family, know the warning signs of toxicity and can be relied upon to stop the drug and report at once. Changes of lithium levels in the blood may occur when a patient switches from mania to depression. A patient with a serum lithium level of 1·0 mmol/l during an attack of mania developed signs of toxicity, and was found to have a serum lithium level of 2·8 mmol/l 10 days after changing to depression, although the oral dosage of lithium remained the same.

Lithium is excreted unchanged through the kidneys, although there is considerable individual variation in renal clearance. Serious renal disease is usually an absolute contraindication to lithium, but patients with lesser degrees of renal impairment can safely be treated with lithium on a lower and more closely monitored dosage. Lithium can be given at any age. Our youngest patient so far is 14 and the oldest 76.

Side effects

These are dose related. One of the most common, and upsetting, is a fine tremor. This is sometimes severe, but can usually be controlled by propranolol, between 10 and 40 mg three times a day. Other side effects include sleepiness, tiredness, nausea, and occasionally vomiting, indigestion and diarrhoea. Thirst is a prominent complaint in about 10 per cent of patients; more than 3 or 4 litres of fluid a day may, in consequence, be drunk and excreted. This 'nephrogenic diabetes insipidus' (NDI) is due to lithium rendering the distal tubules of the kidneys insensitive to the action of antidiuretic hormone, so that water is not reabsorbed. The condition clears up when lithium is stopped.

Oedema of the legs or face can be troublesome, and is presumbaly related to lithium's tendency to retain sodium. Thiazide diuretics can control both the oedema and NDI; but caution is needed when they are combined with lithium, otherwise toxicity may develop. Thiazide results in 24 per cent reduction in renal lithium clearance. It may be advisable to admit the patient requiring a diuretic for a few days to readjust the dosage of lithium. Increase of weight is common and is sometimes the reason for patients stopping lithium. Acne and maculopapular skin eruptions are not uncommon. Psoriasis sometimes becomes worse during lithium treatment.

A benign diffuse goitre is found in a substantial proportion of patients, often with transitory hypothyroidism. This is compensated for by increased TSH and a temporary fall in T4 which soon recovers. Hypothyroidism develops in about 5 per cent of patients, particularly females on long term lithium. It is often necessary to continue lithium, and a combination with thyroxine is satisfactory. Paradoxical cases of hyperthyroidism have also been reported, although these are few and far between. It has been suggested that thyroid function should always be evaluated before starting treatment with lithium and repeated each year. Certainly this is sensible if there is any cause to suspect that hypothyroidism runs in the family.

Changes in the e.c.g. may be seen with non-toxic levels of lithium. Reversible T wave flattening and inversion are most frequent. Bundle branch block can occur. Myocarditis is a rare complication. Manic depressive patients with preexistent arrythmias should be watched carefully; but the evidence to date is that the risks of lithium are far less than the likely benefits in what, after all, is a potentially lethal illness. About one in six patients with manic depression is likely to die by suicide, if untreated.

Rarely a confusional state develops, usually with pre-existing brain damage, in the first 2 or 3 weeks of treatment. Transient neurological abnormalities are sometimes observed, including dysarthria and dysphasia. These neurological complications are more likely when lithium is combined with haloperidol, and other neuroleptics. Although lithium is said to provoke epilepsy in predisposed patients, we have not seen this. All these neurological symptoms clear up rapidly when lithium is stopped.

Signs of toxicity are liable to develop when the serum lithium concentration exceeds 2 mmol/l, but individual patients occasionally develop toxic signs at lower levels. The onset of severe tremor, twitching, nausea, vomiting, anorexia and diarrhoea, slurred speech, unsteadiness and some degree of disorientation, are indications for immediately stopping the drug. Increasing toxicity is followed by oligorenal failure, confusion, fits, coma, and eventually death.

Toxicity is liable to develop in a patient previously stabilised on lithium if

(1) there is cardiac failure,
(2) sodium balance is upset by a low salt diet or a diuretic,
(3) there is increased concentration of lithium when a patient switches rapidly from mania to depression, and
(4) suicide is attempted with lithium overdosage; signs of toxicity only begin to develop several hours after overdosage, and reach a peak after 4 or 5 days.

Lithium crosses the placenta, and concern has been expressed that children of pregnant mothers taking lithium may be at risk; international registers of lithium babies have been set up to monitor this possibility. Lithium is teratogenic in certain animals, but there is no good evidence to date that lithium can damage human babies. But goitre has been reported in the newborn.

Care is required after a woman on lithium has been delivered, since clearance of lithium is greater during pregnancy. Lithium enters breast milk, where its concentration is about one third that of serum. Breast-feeding is probably best avoided; cases of lithium toxicity have been reported in neonates.

Treatment of toxic states

Ideally patients should be nursed in an intensive care unit, where the e.c.g. can be monitored for arrhythmias, respiration maintained, and blood pressure watched. Fits are best treated by intravenous diazepam. Trying to increase excretion of lithium by forced alkaline diuresis probably does more harm than good. Dialysis, both peritoneal and haemodialysis, is effective, but is only required in severe toxic states.

ANTI-PSYCHOTIC DRUGS

For more than a decade before the introduction of neuroleptic drugs a more humane and understanding attitude towards psychotic patients in mental hospitals had been developing. The dangers of institutionalism were recognised, wards were being unlocked, and the concept of the therapeutic community was rapidly spreading. Physical treatments of psychotic patients until 1952 comprised deep insulin therapy, e.c.t. and prefrontal leucotomy. None had specific effects on the vast majority of schizophrenics; two out of three patients admitted to a mental hospital were still there after 2 years.

In 1952 the first neuroleptic drug, reserpine, isolated from the plant rauwolfia, was introduced and found to be effective against schizophrenia. But reserpine had a number of disadvantages, notably a tendency to induce depression, and was rapidly superseded by chlorpromazine; a phenothiazine synthesised during the search for an antihistamine with greater central nervous actions than promethazine. The efficacy of chlorpromazine in psychotic disorders was quickly recognised. Within a few years chlorpromazine, and subsequently other phenothiazines, became the standard treatment for schizophrenia, totally replacing deep insulin therapy. Since 1952, apart from an increasing number of phenothiazine derivatives, other classes of neuroleptic drugs have appeared; thioxanthene derivatives, butyrophenones and diphenylbutylpiperidines. However, none is as satisfactory as the phenothiazines in schizophrenia, which remain the first choice of treatment. Although it is in schizophrenia that the neuroleptics have proved so useful, their actions are also useful in other conditions which cause disturbed behaviour.

Phenothiazine derivatives (See Fig 1.1, p.)

Since the introduction of chlorpromazine, many therapeutically active phenothiazine derivatives have been synthesised; all contain the phenothiazine three-ring structure. They can be divided into three main groups, each characterised by the nature of the side chain substituted on the nitrogen atom in the middle ring (position 10); a dimethyl amino propyl (aliphatic) side chain, i.e. chlorpromazine; a piperidine series, such as thioridazine; and a piperazine group, made up of neuroleptics like trifluoperazine and fluphenazine. All the potent phenothiazines have three methyl groups in their side chain. Individual differences also depend on substitutions made in position 2 (R 1) on the ring; chlorpromazine, for instance, has Cl, trifluoperazine CF3.

The piperazine derivatives are much the most potent, dose for dose (although not necessarily so in clinical efficacy); for instance, 15 mg trifluoperazine is therapeutically equivalent to 300 mg or more of chlorpromazine. The aliphatic and piperidine derivatives have greater anticholinergic properties than the piperazine derivatives, and are therefore less inclined to cause extrapyramidal side effects (see below). All three groups block dopamine receptors and this in turn enhances the release of prolactin from the pituitary, which directly increases the level of prostaglandins. The exact significance of these changes for understanding the action of neuroleptic drugs, and the aetiology of schizophrenia, is still unclear.

Both chlorpromazine and thioridazine are stronger alpha adrenergic receptor blocking agents than piperazine phenothiazines; and in consequence have greater sedative action. Chlorpromazine is therefore preferable to trifluoperazine when agitation and disruptive behaviour are prominent.

The absorption of phenothiazines from the gut varies widely. While some patients absorb chlorpromazine fully and rapidly, others metabolise much of the drug in the wall of the gut or liver before it can enter the blood stream. Obviously in the latter instance, concentration of chlorpromazine in the plasma is low, and may be therapeutically ineffective. Intramuscular and intravenous injections are absorbed directly into the blood stream; they are as much as 50 per cent more effective than phenothiazines given orally.

Phenothiazines are broken down largely in the liver, but their metabolism is complicated and many of their metabolites are themselves therapeutically active. Apart from long-acting preparations, oral phenothiazines require to be given at least twice, and often three times during 24 hours for best effect.

It is particularly in schizophrenic disorders that phenothiazines are so valuable. Schizophrenia remains the major psychosis, at least 6000 new cases—mostly young people—occurring every year in Britain. It is estimated that today there are over 300 000 people in the UK who have had a schizophrenic illness at some time; and that at least one third of them are still receiving treatment, either as impatients, in day centres or hospitals, or at outpatient clinics.

Until the advent of the phenothiazines in 1952, despite the progressively liberal attitudes in mental hospitals in the preceding decades, the number of patients resident there had steadily risen. In the 1950s this was reversed and the mental hospital population began to decline. This was undoubtedly due to the neuroleptic drugs. They quickly abolished acute psychotic symptoms and helped the patient to behave in a socially acceptable manner, and to re-establish communication with others. All this led to the somewhat over-optimistic view that mental hospitals might be unnecessary in the near future.

The pendulum is now beginning to swing back towards commonsense. Neuroleptics can do much, but they cannot cure schizophrenia, and in not a few cases they cannot help at all. Until we discover the cause, or causes of schizophrenia, and they can be remedied, we shall need to protect and provide shelter for many schizophrenics, who simply cannot compete and exist in any reasonable sense outside an 'asylum'.

Nonetheless, we must emphasise again the great therapeutic advances that have occurred as a result of the phenothiazines, the fields of research they have opened up, and in consequence our greater understanding of schizophrenic patients.

Acute schizophrenia presents with highly disturbing symptoms; auditory hallucinations, passivity feelings, and primary delusions, with the patient struggling fearfully to understand what is happening to him, and to regain some sense of control. Most patients need to be treated in hospital at first. This makes their management easier, ensures medication compliance, and that any side effects of neuroleptic drugs are countered. Removing the patient from home, where emotional stresses may be considerable by the time of admission, into the ordered routine of a ward has a calming effect in itself.

Chlorpromazine is first choice for an acutely disturbed patient. It is sensible to keep agitated frightened patients in bed for the first 2 or 3 days after admisssion, well sedated with chlorpromazine, plus a sedative if need be. Three hundred mg a day of chlorpromazine is the minimum required for such a patient, and the daily dose for the first 2 or 3 weeks may need to exceed 1 g. If a patient is unco-operative the dose must be given by injection. Since the whole of the injected dose is absorbed, the dosage is lower than that required by mouth; however the first injection should be in the region of 100 mg to ensure the patient is brought under control as rapidly as possible. When a patient is extremely boisterous it is our practice to give 20 mg haloperidol and 100 mg chlorpromazine by separate injections, and to repeat this if necessary after 2 hours; the most refractory patient usually settles down after this, and is prepared to take medication orally. The sedating effect of chlorpromazine develops at once. Most patients are able to get up after a few days, their anxiety reduced to a tolerable level, ready to trust and accept help from the staff.

When chlorpromazine is contraindicated, for instance when there is a history of an allergic response such as jaundice during previous treatment, or the patient has serious liver damage, thioridazine can be employed. But it is not as effective, and the dosage must not exceed 800 mg a day; with higher doses retinopathy is a risk.

It usually takes 1 to 2 weeks before the antipsychotic action of the drug manifests itself. Once the patient begins to improve, the dosage of phenothiazine should be reduced to a level which is still effectively antipsychotic, yet has minimal side effects. However, it is advisable to maintain a patient on at least 300 mg a day of, for instance, chlorpromazine for the first fortnight of treatment. Too early reduction allows psychotic symptoms to reappear.

Some patients dislike the sedating effect of chlorpromazine, and prefer a piperazine phenothiazine such as trifluoperazine; 15 mg a day in three divided doses is equivalent to around 300 mg of chlorpromazine. Extrapyramidal side effects are particularly common with the piperazine group, and dystonic reactions are frightening and painful. It is important not to misinterpret these as schizophrenic or hysterical symptoms, and to give an antiParkinsonian drug at once parenterally.

Patients with paranoid schizophrenia, particularly those whose symptoms develop in middle age or later, tend to be less agitated and disturbed than young acutely ill patients. Trifluoperazine suits them better than chlorpromazine, in a dosage of between 15 and 30 mg a day at first, and certainly trifluoperazine is more suitable for psychotics of 70 years or older, liable to develop troublesome postural hypotension and confusion on large doses of chlorpromazine.

The average time an acute schizophrenic patient spends in our unit, on his first admission, is 6 weeks. Rehabilitation begins as soon as he is up and about; he attends OT and takes part in ward activities and group meetings. But care must be taken not to put too much emotional pressure on him. Psychotherapy of an interpretative kind should be avoided. He must be helped to deal with the stresses at home or work which may have contributed to his illness. And it is usually necessary to see relatives, advise them, and enlist their co-operation. Important decisions about when a patient can return to work, when a housewife is ready to look after her family again, if a student is likely to return to university, must be made. The patient may benefit from vocational training schemes, a protected job arranged through the Disablement Resettlement Officer, and sometimes by living away from home in a special hostel. Indeed, the greatest skill in helping many schizophrenics comes after the patient has left hospital.

It was quickly appreciated that phenothiazines did not cure schizophrenia, and that many patients relapsed when they stopped medication. For instance, in 1959, 42 per cent of schizophrenics discharged from mental hospitals in London relapsed and needed readmission within 1 year. By contrast, only 18 per cent of similar patients in Edinburgh relapsed. The difference was due to poor follow-up in London and, in consequence, the patients no longer taking their medication. More recent studies have confirmed that phenothiazines protect many schizophrenics from relapsing.

The introduction of long-acting phenothiazine and thioxanthene preparation has made the treatment of chronic schizophrenic states much simpler. Regular injections of fluphenazine decanoate, or flupenthixol decanoate, every 2 to 4 weeks, ensure that the neuroleptic is fully absorbed. Drug defaulting is kept of a minimum, for a close check can be kept on each patient's attendance; if he fails to keep his appointment he can be visited at home. This has the additional advantage of exposing emotional problems not previously suspected. It is now well known that a major cause of a schizophrenic's relapse lies in the nature of his environment. A home where there is too much overtly expressed criticism or overprotective emotion is likely to lead to the re-emergence of acute psychotic symptoms. Brown and his colleagues have demonstrated clearly the importance of such factors as face-to-face contact in a critical atmosphere; relapse is probable when this exceeds 35 hours a week.

A phenothiazine protects a patient by allowing him to tolerate more emotional strain than he could otherwise do. The drug thereby enlarges the patient's life and allows him to function better socially. Before the era of neuroleptics, the schizophrenic had to withdraw and cut himself off emotionally from other people to avoid relapse. Studies have shown that, without the cover of a neuroleptic, 9 out of 10 schizophrenics going from hospital to homes of high 'expressed emotion' are likely to relapse within 9 months. This rate falls to 50 per cent when the patient receives regular medication; and to about half as much again if the environment can also be controlled and high levels of emotion and criticism avoided. It is important to recognise that tensions at home are often the result of a patient's symptoms and difficult behaviour, and that when these are controlled by neuroleptics emotional confrontations decline. However the converse is also harmful. A home which lacks stimulation allows the schizophrenic to sink into an inert withdrawn state; the 'institutionalised' condition seen so often in the chronic wards of mental hospitals 50 years ago.

The majority of recovered schizophrenics need to continue neuroleptic medication for several years, perhaps indefinitely, but not all do. Comparisons of long-acting neuroleptics with a placebo in cases of chronic schizophrenia have demonstrated that 66 per cent of patients given the placebo relapse over the period of 1 year. But it is as well to note that one third do not. Some of these may live emotionally quiet lives. In time a much greater proportion would probably relapse. However, clearly it is wrong to cast a therapeutic blanket over schizophrenia; each patient must be considered separately. There is no reason to doubt that many schizophrenics can exist satisfactorily for long periods without maintenance drug therapy.

It seems generally agreed that simple schizophrenics, and 'burnt out' schizophrenics with little capacity for emotional feeling, do not benefit from receiving a neuroleptic regularly. Treatment with a phenothiazine merely takes away what little drive and affect may be left, with no advantage to the patient.

Many patients who suffer an acute schizo-affective or schizophreniform illness recover fully and have no further attack. Clearly, if this is so, it is unnecessary to continue with a neuroleptic after they have recovered. The problem is the perennial one of diagnosis. But faced with a first time illness, which developed acutely in someone of previously outgoing personality, precipitated by some stressful event, and strongly coloured by depression or confusion, it is reasonable, after the condition has fully subsided, to stop treatment. Obviously, a family history of relapsing or chronic schizophrenia must raise doubts, and in such cases it may be advisable to continue the neuroleptic for a year or so after recovery, while observing the patient's progress. In any case, if the patient is returning to university, has an important examination to pass, or promotion is at hand, it may be better to play for safety and give a phenothiazine until the hurdle is passed. Of course, if a patient relapses when off medication, maintenance therapy is then a necessity.

How long a neuroleptic needs to be continued depends on numerous factors, most of which have been discussed above. Each patient's needs must be asssessed individually, not least the consequences to his working and social life if he relapses. A minimum of 3 years' maintenance treatment for most schizophrenics is advisable, and the drug is only stopped then if the patient has remained free of symptoms during this time.

Other indications for phenothiazine derivatives

1. Mania. Before neuroleptics were available, mania was a most difficult condition to treat, requiring padded cells and forced feeding in its extreme forms; the mortality rate for acute mania was high. Today most cases of mania can be controlled rapidly; but difficult patients may take a week or so to calm, and e.c.t. is still occasionally needed.

Acute mania usually responds to large doses of chlorpromazine, up to 2 g a day initially. Frequently it is impossible to give the drug orally and the parenteral route must be used; 100 to 200 mg chlorpromazine intramuscularly is painful but effective. A few patients remain extremely difficult to control. If a combination of 100 mg chlorpromazine with 20 mg haloperidol is given intravenously and repeated if need be after 1 to 2 hours, control is gained immediately. Once the patient falls asleep chlorpromazine and /or haloperidol are given just frequently enough to ensure that he remains drowsy, yet able to eat and drink adequately. After 4 or 5 days the most difficult patient begins to return to normality.

Lithium is of course the most specific treatment available. If a manic patient is prepared to take drugs orally, lithium can be started at once (provided there is no doubt about the diagnosis). There is little point in giving heroic doses of 2 g or more a day, as Cade did in 1947, for lithium takes at least 10 to 14 days before its effects are felt; it is better to rely on chlorpromazine and/or haloperidol for immediate calming effects.

2. Depression. Phenothiazine derivatives can be combined with antidepressant drugs. It is suggested that they potentiate antidepressants by inhibiting their breakdown in the liver. Chlorpromazine is invaluable in severely agitated depression; up to 300 mg a day together with amitriptyline and e.c.t., may be needed for a time. Hypotension is the only troublesome effect of this combination.

A piperazine phenothiazine such as trifluoperazine is useful in depressive paranoid states; between 5 and 15 mg a day can be combined with the antidepressant.

On their own, phenothiazine derivatives have no specific antidepressant action. But many agitated and anxious patients, particularly those past middle age, respond well to small doses of a piperazine phenothiazines alone; say 1 to 2 mg of trifluoperzine, two or three times a day. They have the additional advantage in old patients of not causing hypotension.

3. Toxic confusional states. Many respond well to neuroleptic drugs. Chlorpromazine is indicated when a patient is severely agitated, following for instance the ingestion of hallucinogenic or amphetamine drugs. Delirium tremens may require large doses of chlorpromazine, but serious liver damage is a contraindication, and the risk of fits is high; chlormethiazole and lorazepam are, in the main, better drugs for delirium tremens. Barbiturate withdrawal is best managed by progressively reducing the dosage of barbiturate, with the protection of a diazepam derivative; as in delirium tremens, the risk of epileptic fits is increased by chlorpromazine. The anxiety and agitation that may accompany or follow surgical operations, admission to a coronary care unit, or even to a hospital ward, often respond best to a small dose of a piperazine phenothiazine, or haloperidol.

4. Neurotic states (including anorexia nervosa). Small doses of a neuroleptic are occasionally better than tranquillisers in alleviating neurotic anxiety. A piperazine phenothiazine 1 to 2 mg a day, or haloperidol 0·5 mg, two or three times a day, is particularly effective in reducing the anxiety and agitated behaviour that is so common in old age. Depression is not prominent in many of these patients. Antidepressant drugs readily cause confusion and diazepine derivatives sometimes seem to make these patients worse.

Their use in combination with antidepressant drugs has already been mentioned. The combination of a piperazine phenothiazine with a MAOI is particularly effective in relieving symptoms of atypical depression. But when cardiovascular symptoms such as palpitations and tachycardia are prominent a diazepine derivative is usually better. Caution is needed when prescribing neuroleptics to young people, for dystonic reactions are particularly common.

Chlorpromazine or thioridazine, taken an hour before bedtime, may help obsessionally anxious patients to get to sleep and remain so until morning, even without a hypnotic drug. The dose varies from 25 to 100 mg, but large amounts are liable to cause hangover effects.

Chlorpromazine still has a place in the inpatient treatment of anorexia nervosa (see Ch. 00), and small doses, from 10 to 25 mg three times a day, can relax those tense, obsessional/hysterical middle-aged women who are perennially underweight, and express their disatisfactions towards those on whom they depend by not eating enough to maintain weight; small amounts of a tricyclic antidepressant usually need to be given in addition.

5. *Aggressive behaviour,* from whatever cause, which fails to respond to firm but sympathetic and patient handling, can be controlled rapidly by neuroleptics. Since the patient is likely to be unco-operative, the drugs must be given intramuscularly; this has the advantage of the whole dose being rapidly absorbed. Small patients, who are unco-operative rather than dangerously violent, are given chlorpromazine 50 to 100 mg, or haloperidol 10 mg, repeated every 1 to 2 hours depending on the response.

Side effects

Central nervous system. All the phenothiazines are capable of sedation in large enough dosage, and all have additive effects with hypnotics and sedatives. About 15 per cent of treated patients become depressed; but long acting phenothiazines have no greater tendency in this respect than other phenothiazines. Rarely, a state of excitement with aggressive paranoid behaviour develops soon after starting treatment. Toxic confusional states are unusual, and occur mainly in the elderly.

Extrapyramidal syndromes may develop with any of the potent neuroleptics, even with a minute dose, although these are more likely after large ones; those commonly seen are Parkinsonism, dyskinesia and akathisia. These side effects result from the balance between dopamine and acetylcholine in the brain being disturbed. Neuroleptics with strong anticholinergic properties, such as thioridazine, are less likely to produce Parkinsonism. The piperazine derivatives are the worst offenders. There is no evidence to substantiate earlier claims that antipsychotic and extrapyramidal effects necessarily go hand in hand.

Parkinsonism and akathisia are the commonest, dystonic the most frightening reactions. Dystonic reactions develop within 2 to 3 days of starting treatment, and are particularly likely to occur in young patients, and those with hysterical personalities.

Tardive dyskinesia affects usually the mouth, tongue and face and tends to develop when a neuroleptic is given for a long period; but the phenomenon can occur after only a few months of high dosage. Pre-existent brain damage may render a patient more prone to this side effect. It is not yet possible to anticipate which patient may develop tardive dyskinesia, and it is important therefore always to be on watch for its signs. The condition may worsen if the neuroleptic is suddenly stopped. Nonetheless, the majority of patients gradually improve when the drug is stopped, although this can take up to a year. But sometimes signs persist indefinitely or even increase and it may then be necessary to restart the neuroleptic; signs and symptoms then disappear. It may, of course, be impossible in any event to stop the drug without worsening the psychosis. AntiParkinsonian drugs have no effect on tardive dyskinesia.

AntiParkinsonian drugs are sometimes prescribed routinely with a neuroleptic. This is bad practice, for antiParkinsonian drugs themselves can produce side effects, and may reduce the absorption of phenothiazines from the gut. They can also antagonise a neuroleptic's anti-psychotic activity and they may increase the risk of tardive dyskinesia. It is reasonable to prescribe them at the start of treatment to avoid possible dystonic reactions, but after a fortnight they should be slowly withdrawn, and only continued if extrapyramidal signs appear. Less than a third of schizophrenics maintained on phenothiazines need antiParkinsonian drugs.

Automatic nervous dysfunction. Anticholinergic and alpha-adrenoceptor blocking effects are responsible for such side effects as dry mouth, constipation, blurred vision, tachycardia, and postural hypotension. Urinary retention is occasionally troublesome, and sexual dysfunction upsetting.

Cardiovascular effects. Changes in the e.c.g., particularly abnormal T-waves, often occur especially with thioridazine. Ventricular tachycardia is a rare complication, and is occasionally fatal; this usually follows overdose.

Allergic reactions. Cholestatic jaundice is an uncommon complication of chlorpromazine, and is an idiocyncratic reaction, occurring in the first 3 months of treatment. Jaundice seemed to be much more prevalent when the drug was first introduced. It is now quite a rare reaction. If jaundice develops chlorpromazine should be stopped and another phenothiazine substituted.

Agranulocytosis is a very rare toxic effect of chlorpromazine and thioridazine. It does not occur with the piperazine phenothiazines.

Endocrine changes. Women given prolonged treatment with a phenothiazine are liable to develop prolactinaemia, which causes galactorrhoea and amenorrhoea. Gynaecomastia is occasionally seen in men.

Skin changes. Photosensitivity is common with chlorpromazine, and patients should always be warned of the dangers of sunshine. Skin rashes of a maculopapular kind, are most likely to follow chlorpromazine. Melanin is deposited in areas of exposed skin when phenothiazines are given for long periods; this causes a brownish pigmentation.

The eye. Deposits of melanin may also appear in the cornea and lens. Retinitis pigmentosa is a danger with thioridazine when more than 800 mg a day is given for a prolonged period.

Miscellaneous effects. Oedema, which is rarely severe, is most likely with chlorpromazine; it is a common side effect during treatment of anorexia nervosa.

Weight gain is sometimes considerable, and patients may have great difficulty in dieting and losing weight while on a phenothiazine.

Thioxanthene derivatives

With the thioxanthene derivatives the central ring has been modified by replacing the nitrogen atom with one of carbon. Exactly the same substitutions at R1 and R2 can be made as in the phenothiazine derivatives.

The thioxanthene derivatives are less potent, dose for dose, than the phenothiazines, and by and large less effective. However, flupenthixol seems to be comparable to fluphenazine in clinical effectiveness. Both are used as long-acting neuroleptics. Forty mg flupenthixol decanoate is equivalent to 25 mg fluphenazine decanoate. Flupenthixol is claimed to have an antidepressant effect but this is misleading. The drug does, however, tend to have a less lowering effect on mood and drive than fluphenazine. We prefer flupenthixol to fluphenazine when affect is good; fluphenazine when there is a possibility of aggressive impulsive behaviour. Intramuscular injections are needed every 1 to 4 weeks.

Smaller doses of flupenthixol, 10 to 20 mg at 2 to 3 weekly intervals can occasionally help patients other than psychotics to control their impulses; alcoholic binges, outbursts of destructive anger, psychopathic behaviour and so on. We have on several occasions found the combination of 20 mg flupenthixol intramuscularly fortnightly with tranylcypromine orally to be most effective in helping patients with pathological jealousy, arising out of an insecure personality. Treatment must be continued for at least 6 months in order to allow psychotherapy time to make adequate headway.

Small doses of flupenthixol by mouth are claimed to lift depression. Some neurotic states of depression do respond to the drug, but it is in no way a substitute for the tricyclic and MAOI groups of antidepressants.

Butyrophenones and variations

Haloperidol is the prototype of the butyrophenones. All are potent inhibitors of dopamine. They have little or no anticholinergic or adrenoceptor blocking effects. Haloperidol is rapidly absorbed from the gut, and reaches a plasma peak within 40 minutes. When given intramuscularly the peak plasma level is attained within 20 minutes. Excretion is slow and cumulative effects develop when more than two doses a day are given. The half-life varies between 15 and 22 hours. Haloperidol can be given orally, intramuscularly or intravenously.

Haloperidol is used to control mania and hypomania, catatonic excitement, and acute confusional states; indeed, it is useful for treating any seriously disturbed patient. Treatment starts with 10 to 15 mg a day or more orally, and is increased until the patient's behaviour quietens. Up to 100 mg a day may be required for a time. Once the patient improves the dosage is gradually reduced.

Manic depression, only partially controlled by lithium, may need the addition of haloperidol to control up swings. Although haloperidol and lithium have been successfully combined for many years, reports have recently suggested that toxic effects may accrue; in one reported case the patient was left with permanent brain damage. We ourselves have had two patients who developed toxic symptoms while taking both drugs, which disappeared within 24 hours of stopping lithium. The combination is certainly not contraindicated in our view, but it does require clinical care and circumspection.

In difficult cases intramuscular or intravenous routes are necessary. Rapid 'neuroleptisation' involves giving 10 mg of haloperidol intramuscularly every half hour; six injections are usually enough. Once control is gained, oral haloperidol is substituted.

Chronic schizophrenics, resistent to phenothiazines, provided they are not emotionally deteriorated, may respond well to high dose therapy, with up to 200 mg haloperidol a day. This is reduced as improvement occurs. Longstanding auditory hallucinations, particularly those associated with alcoholism, disappear within a week or so of starting haloperidol, when other neuroleptics may not have helped.

Small doses of haloperidol, 1 to 3 mg a day, are useful as an anxiolytic, especially in old people, and 1·5 mg is a safe hypnotic. Claims have been made for haloperidol in the treatment of motor tics, stuttering and childhood behaviour problems. The Gilles de la Tourette syndrome, of tics and coprolalia, seems to respond specifically to haloperidol, whatever the age of the patient.

Given intravenously with an anaesthetic, 10 mg haloperidol lessens the risk of confusion and agitation following e.c.t. Haloperidol is usually given twice a day, but Ayd claims that a single dose, given at night, is enough in chronic psychotic states.

Side effects are minimal apart from extrapyramidal symptoms, and the incidence of these is much the same as with the piperazine phenothiazines. AntiParkinsonian drugs are required in about 50 per cent of patients on medium dosage, but high dosage and parenteral injections rarely cause extrapyramidal side effects. The drug is remarkably safe, but tardive dyskinesia must be watched for when treatment is prolonged.

Other derivations include triperidol, which seems to have no particular advantage over haloperidol, droperidol and benperidol; the latter lessens sexual libido, and is sometimes used in the treatment of sexual offenders.

Diphenylbutylpiperidines.
Substitutions, particularly in the phenylpiperidine part of the molecule, provide a group of diphenylbutylpiperidines; pimozide, penfluridol, fluspiriline. These drugs all have an exceptionally long action, and the risk of extrapyramidal side effects is less than with haloperidol or piperazine phenothiazines. All block dopamine receptors.

Pimozide need be taken once a day only. Oral dosage in the treatment of schizophrenia ranges from 10 to 20 mg or more a day. Smaller doses are used for neurotic states of anxiety, in the same way as haloperidol. Claims that pimozide is especially effective in hypochondriasis are of the anecdotal kind.

Side effects are few, but skin rashes occasionally occur. Depression may be increased, as with any dopamine blocker. Agitation sometimes becomes worse, and pimozide is best avoided when this is present.

Penfluridol, in a dose of 30 mg, is given orally, and acts for about a week. The drug enters and leaves the brain very slowly.

Fluspirilene, 1 to 10 mg intramuscularly, has a duration of action of about a week, with a peak effect after 2 days.

These drugs are used in chronic schizophrenia unresponsive to phenothiazines and other neuroleptics, or for patients particularly prone to develop extrapyramidal side effects.

ANXIOLYTICS AND HYPNOTICS

Anxiety develops whenever we feel ourselves threatened. The threat may be a real one, and concern a man's job or his marriage, or disgrace and loss of self esteem. But often the threat arises mainly from within a patient, from his basic sense of insecurity.

Anxiety, up to a point, is useful; it makes an individual alert and ready for action, and narrows his attention onto the threat, but when anxiety becomes too great it ceases to be of benefit. The sufferer becomes indecisive, and his behaviour maladaptive, even bizarre. He is incapable of facing his problems. He may attempt to run away, but is frozen to the spot, like a rabbit before a stoat.

Anxiety can involve virtually every system in the body; ultimately, a patient may come to focus all his anxiety onto physical symptoms, convinced that he has a brain tumour, leukaemia, heart disease, multiple sclerosis and such like. He may in fact have hypertension and ischaemic heart disease, chronic bronchitis, or an irritable colon, and his fears may build themselves around these conditions. Very frequently he displaces his fears onto some external situation, thereby shutting out the real cause of his anxiety; he becomes afraid to travel by public transport, or to eat in a restaurant, to sign his name in front of others, to go into a crowded shop. Eventually he may become completely housebound.

Anxiety states like these may continue long after the original cause of anxiety has been removed, fear feeding on fear, creating a perpetually expanding vicious circle. Anxiety may of course be secondary to schizophrenia or depression; depression without anxiety in attendance is exceptional. Anxiety also arises in the early stages of dementia, while insight is still retained.

Treatment of an anxiety state requires the fullest understanding of a patient, his personality and constitution, the problems lying behind his anxiety, and the consequences, including any possible gains, if symptoms continue. A man of stable personality, well able to deal with his problems in the past, may only require to discuss his fears with someone sympathetic and sensible in order to recover. But he may also require a hypnotic for a week or two, to stop him ruminating on his troubles after retiring to bed, and to ensure a good 7 to 8 hours sleep. When anxiety has been present for many months and the patient is worn out by his symptoms, a tranquilliser will give him fresh courage to face his difficulties. If signs of reactive depression have begun to appear he may benefit from a MAOI combined with the tranquilliser. Psychotherapy needs to be geared to a patients's needs; the constitutional neurotic may well require more prolonged and deeper interpretation of his anxieties than the reasonably phlegmatic man. Behaviour therapy may be needed, particularly when phobic symptoms are evident, and is likely to be most successful when the original cause of anxiety has disappeared.

Drugs, including alcohol and tobacco, have always had an important part to play in combating human anxiety. Opium was widely used until its addictive properties forced its restriction by legislation. There are still a number of chronic anxiety neurotics dependent on chlorodyne. Bromides were popular before the barbiturates and were undoubtedly effective, but their tendency to cause a toxic state—bromism—especially in older patients, was a disadvantage, and has now led to their almost complete withdrawal.

Barbiturates

The barbiturates have been in use since the start of this century. They reached their prescription peak about 10 years ago. They exert a generalised depressant effect on the nervous system, particularly the neocortex and reticular formation. They are still widely used as hypnotics. At present they are denounced for causing dependence and serious withdrawal symptoms, including fits, disturbing the sleeping e.e.g., interacting adversely with other drugs, and for providing an easy means of suicide. While no one will deny that they have great disadvantages, the barbiturates are unexcelled in acute anxiety, and as hypnotics for some insomniacs; there are patients who waken refreshed after a night's sleep with 100 mg butobarbitone, yet feel dull and headachy after a benzodiazepine hypnotic. And many a phobic patient is still reassured by the knowledge that he carries with him 50 mg quinalbarbitone for emergencies.

Phenobarbitone causes and enhances depression, and should not be used for psychiatric syndromes. Barbiturates are particularly likely to cause confusion in elderly patients. They are contraindicated in patients with porphyria.

Intravenous sodium amylobarbitone is still valuable in psychiatric emergencies. An acutely anxious patient, panic-striken and hysterical, who has recently been subjected to some appalling misfortune—a car or rail crash, a gang rape, her husband killed before her eyes—needs to be rapidly and heavily sedated, and allowed to sleep for 12 hours or more at a stretch. Intravenous sodium amylobarbitone, 250 to 500 mg produces deep sleep immediately. Once asleep, chlorpromazine or a diazepine can be given intramuscularly to ensure that sleep is prolonged. The patient wakens refreshed and sufficiently calm to discuss what has happened and what has to be done. Diazepine derivatives, by mouth or parenterally, have nothing like the same effect.

Smaller doses of sodium amylobarbitone, or the shorter acting pentobarbitone or methohexitone, are used to relax a tense inhibited patient and help her to discuss problems and events in her life which she would otherwise have difficulty in disclosing (see p. 79). The same technique can be used in hysterical conversion. A small dose of barbiturate is slowly injected intravenously; hysterical amnesia or paralysis quickly disappear. It is then of vital importance to discover the cause, and to deal with the patient's anxiety, which develops immediately dissociation lifts.

Barbiturates, with the exception of barbitone, are broken down in the liver by microsomal enzymes, and in the process the activity of these enzymes is increased. As a result, other drugs metabolised by them, tricyclic antidepressants and phenothiazines for example, are broken down more rapidly. Barbiturates also interact with coumarin anticoagulants.

Their rapid withdrawal from a patient anticoagulated with warfarin is potentially hazardous.

Benzodiazepine derivatives

This group of drugs appeared in the early 1960s and has now largely replaced barbiturates and meprobamate. Benzodiazepines are less likely to cause tolerance and physical dependence, are less sedating, and are safe even after huge overdoses. They do not interact appreciably with other drugs, and they do not influence the activity of liver microsomal enzymes responsible for metabolising other drugs. Their mode of action is still unclear, but is thought to involve the limbic system (where emotional feelings are aroused by and attached to incoming information), the reticular activating system and the hypothalamus. They probably influence neurotransmitters, but evidence to date is contradictory. They are metabolised in the liver, and some of their metabolites are themselves active.

The benzodiazepines reduce anxiety without an uncomfortable degree of sedation; there are differences in this respect between diazepine compounds, related to their half-life and metabolites. Their sedative effect increases with dosage, and large doses are used to counter insomnia. Many of them relax voluntary muscles. Muscle tone is usually increased in anxiety states, and the muscle relaxation induced by these drugs may in itself reduce anxiety. Some, such as diazepam and clonazepam, are effective as anticonvulsants.

Their main use is in the treatment of anxiety, however severe. Even when anxiety is secondary to depression or schizophrenia, a benzodiazepine can be of benefit, combined of course with the appropriate antidepressant or neuroleptic. Numerous trials of benzodiazepines against other anxiolytics, placebo, and between benzodiazepine derivatives themselves, have been reported; the majority confirm that all the benzodiazepines are clinically active. So far as the different diazepines are concerned, there is probably little difference in their anxiolytic power. But they do differ in their half-lives and metabolism; diazepam for instance has a comparatively long half-life, and is metabolised largely to desmethyldiazepam, which itself is active and has a very long half-life. Oxazepam and lorazepam on the other hand, have a shortish half-life and none of their metabolites is active; there is therefore less likelihood of accumulation. The benzodiazepines are also widely used as hypnotics; nitrazepam and flurazepam are probably the most popular, but in fact any of the group has a hypnotic effect if given in high enough dosage.

The value of diazepines in the treatment of alcohol withdrawal is increasingly being recognised. Delirium tremens can be controlled more effectively than by any other compound, including chlormethiazole. We prefer lorazepam, (see Ch. 11), because its shorter action allows better control of the patient; the dosage can be readily adjusted to give the required level of sedation, and side effects are minimal. The diazepines also have the advantage of lessening the likelihood of fits.

Diazepam and lorazepam can be given intravenously, as an emergency measure in panic attacks, with the anaesthetic in e.c.t., as an aid to behaviour therapy, and to control status epilepticus. Either can be used as an anaesthetic in minor operations and techniques, where their ability to induce amnesia is often an advantage.

Chlordiazepoxide was the first of the group to be introduced for the control of anxiety. Its value was immediately recognised and it quickly began to replace meprobamate and the barbiturates. It was followed by diazepam, and subsequently by a number of other compounds. Diazepam is preferred by many patients with chronic anxiety, partly because its anxiolytic effects are felt more rapidly; presumably because absorption is quicker. Diazepam is also liable to cause a greater degree of sedation than chlordiazepoxide, unless only very small doses are given. Of course, if chlordiazepoxide is given in high dosage, say 75 mg or more a day, sedation becomes apparent.

Acute anxiety, where some sedative effect is desirable, is better treated with diazepam than a shorter lasting analogue. All the diazepines can be combined safely with other drugs, although it is important to recognise that they potentiate alcohol and sedative drugs. Chlormethiazole and benzodiazepines potentiate one another's effects powerfully; dangerously when alcohol is also present.

Tachycardia, palpitation, and tremor, are often major complaints of patients with anxiety; anxiety is increasingly focussed onto these symptoms and a vicious circle effect ensues. Propranolol on its own can often block these symptoms, with some lift in anxiety, but it is the combination of propranolol , 20 to 40 mg three times a day, with diazepam 5 mg three times day, which can sometimes produce such dramatic improvement in these patients.

Anxiety often improves after starting a diazepine, but the patient may then complain of feeling depressed. It is unlikely that the drug has caused depression. Rather, the clinician has overlooked the presence of depression underlying anxiety symptoms. It is now that the combination of a diazepine with a MAOI, such a phenelzine or tranylcypromine, is so effective (see p. 20).

The dosage of commonly used diazepines is shown in Table 1·3. There is considerable individual variation to the same dose. It is advisable to start the treatment of a patient who is moderately anxious with a smallish dose and increase slowly, depending on the patient's reaction; for example 2 mg diazepam two or three times a day, and perhaps 5 mg an

Table 1.3 Dosage of diazepines

Diazepine	Average daily dose	Average bedtime dose	Larger daily doses used for short periods
Diazepam	2–5 mg t.d.s.	5–10 mg	120 mg
Chlordiazepoxide	5–10 mg t.d.s.	10–25 mg	600 mg
Oxazepam	10–15 mg t.d.s.	15–30 mg	120 mg
Lorazepam	1–2·5 mg t.d.s.	2·5–5 mg	25 mg
Clobazam	10 mg t.d.s.	10–20 mg	60 mg
Medazepam	5–10 mg t.d.s.	10–20 mg	60 mg
Potassium chlorazepate	—	15 mg	45 mg
Flurazepam	—	15–30 mg	150 mg
Nitrazepam	—	5–10 mg	25 mg

hour or so before bedtime, doubling or even trebling this over the space of the next 2 weeks if need be. With more severe anxiety, particularly if a patient is off work and does not have to drive a car, treatment can begin with 10 mg three times day and 20 mg at night. Occasionally speed of action is indicated, or a patient may refuse or be unable to take the drug orally; for instance in delirium tremens. The diazepine must then be given by injection. Most of the analogues can be given intramuscularly, although this can be a painful process. Only diazepam and lorazepam may be given intravenously.

A patient in a state of panic responds well to intravenous diazepam, 10 to 20 mg. An intramuscular injection may be needed to produce sleep in a hospitalised patient; 100 mg of chloridazepoxide, or 20 to 30 mg diazepam is usually adequate. For the patient in delirium tremens the dose may need to be repeated every 2 or 3 hours for a day or so.

Benzodiazepines, like other effective anxiolytics and sedatives, are liable to be abused by both patient and doctor. Many practitioners are all too ready to prescribe a benzodiazepine for minor complaints, for anxiety which is understandable and in no way incapacitating, or without recognising the psychotic disorder underlying the anxiety. Inadequate patients with chronic anxiety may slowly build up tolerance and dependence, although this is rare compared to other sedatives, until they are ingesting very large amounts indeed. One man, who obtained his supplies from several practitioners, was eventually taking between 150 and 250 mg diazepam a day; under such conditions it was no wonder that he described his life as 'peaceful'.

Many anxious patients do need to continue with diazepam for a long time, perhaps indefinitely; some regularly, others intermittently. It is sometimes difficult to know whether or when to wean a patient off his drug, for he may object strongly to the removal of what he has come to see as a necessary crutch. How forceful the doctor should be depends largely on the patient's circumstances and personality, but in any event, he should not continue to prescribe without periodically reviewing the patient's case.

When a patient has been on a benzodiazepine for many months, the drug must not be stopped abruptly; otherwise anxiety may return and withdrawal effects appear. These are much less serious than those following barbiturate or meprobamate withdrawal; they develop over 2 or 3 days and may continue for a week or more unless the drug is resumed.

Side effects are remarkably few. Drowsiness and tiredness occur with too high a dosage, particularly those drugs with long lives and active metabolites. At the start of treatment patients must always be warned of this possibility and cautioned to take care when driving. They must also know that the effects of alcohol and other sedative drugs, and antihistamines, are additive. Ataxia is only likely to develop on large doses. Some patients gain a considerable amount of weight. Occasionally, and mainly in old people, these drugs cause confusion and alarming visual hallucinations. Rarely a 'paradoxical reaction' develops soon after starting a benzodiazepine; the patient becomes angry and aggressive. For the most part these drugs have the opposite effect.

Some patients complain of impairment of recent memory, that they become forgetful and absent-minded when taking a benzodiazepine. Certainly, amnesia may be complete for up to 30 minutes after intravenous diazepam.

These drugs cross the placenta and build up to a concentration in the foetus comparable to that in the mother. They may have teratogenic effects. There have been occasional reports of an increased incidence of hare lip, sometimes associated with cleft palate, in the children of mothers given diazepam during pregnancy.

Contraindications. Benzodiazepines, like other sedatives, should be avoided in respiratory failure. In liver failure, only short-acting diazepines such as oxazepam or lorazepam should be given. They should be avoided in pregnancy, if possible. Caution is needed with unstable patients liable to develop tolerance and become dependent.

Hypnotics

Our understanding of sleep and its functions has greatly increased over the past 20 years, thanks to sleeping e.e.g. studies. There are five e.e.g. stages. When a person first falls asleep he passes almost at once to stage 4 NREM, the deepest stage. After a variable time he moves back through the different stages until, after 60 to 90 minutes, he reaches the stage which coincides with rapid eye movements (REM) and vivid dreams; these are readily recalled if the subject is woken. The REM stage at this point in sleep may last for only a few minutes, and gradually gives way again to deep non REM sleep (NREM). During an average night's sleep, of 7 to 8 hours, there are about four of these cycles. In all, the REM stage takes up about 25 per cent of total sleep.

REM sleep seems to be necessary for the restoration of mental functions, NREM sleep for the repair of body tissues. Although patients can manage with indefinitely suppressed REM sleep, with phenelzine say, prevention of REM sleep by physical arousal builds up to produce a rebound phenomenon, greatly prolonged periods of REM sleep, until the deficiency is restored. If sleep is totally prevented for 48 hours or more, hallucinations develop. 5HT may play some part in this. It is certainly important for sleep; when the concentration of 5HT is low insomnia occurs, and REM sleep in particular is reduced.

Although vivid, easily recallable dreaming develops only in the REM stage, dreaming probably occurs at all levels, including stage 4 NREM, although it is then difficult to recall. Childhood night terrors arise in stage 4 sleep, whereas nightmares develop during REM sleep. Sleep-walking is associated with stage 4.

The prolonged use of most hypnotics interferes with REM sleep at first, but gradually this is re-established; there is still a marked rebound when the drugs are stopped. Nightmares and vivid dreams then abound, waking the patient and disrupting his sleep, and often requiring the hypnotic to be resumed.

Insomnia has many causes. Difficulty in getting to sleep may be due to pain, when an analgesic is then preferable to a hypnotic, a strange and uncomfortable bed, air travel disrupting the biological rhythm, or strong coffee and stimulating drugs taken too late in the day. Anxious patients, although tired, begin to churn over the days events as soon as they close their eyes. The more they try to stop their thoughts, the more remote sleep becomes. Even when they fall asleep they may immediately be woken by hypnogogic hallucinations. People with obsessional personalities become obsessed with the need for 'proper' sleep, and so tense when they fail to fall asleep instantly that insomnia is prolonged. In such cases a benzodiazepine taken an hour or so before bedtime may reduce tension and obsessional thinking sufficiently to induce sleep. Alternatively, such patients can be 'knocked out' when in bed by chloral hydrate 1 to 2 g; still a most useful drug, its main disadvantages being its taste, and dependency in patients with addictive personalities.

With increasing age the amount of sleep needed diminishes. After middle age sleeping is often erratic, the individual waking several times at night. A heavy drinker is also liable to waken after 4 or 5 hours sleep, with frightening dreams if serious withdrawal effects are developing. Waking after 4 or 5 hours is also a characteristic and early symptom of endogenous depression, usually accompanied by a sense of apprehension and despair. If this is the cause of insomnia, a suitable antidepressant drug must be started without delay. The sedating tricyclic antidepressants, such as trimipramine and amitriptyline can be given in a single dose at bedtime, and may be enough to combat insomnia. But often a hypnotic needs to be combined with them.

Anxious patients, particularly those faced with a serious problem about which they are uncertain and indecisive, are liable to dream vividly enough to wake themselves several times during the night. If the problem is likely to be resolved within a week or so, a hypnotic which suppresses REM sleep and vivid dreaming is helpful. If it is only required for a few days, a barbiturate, 100 pentobarbitone say, is ideally suited for the purpose.

Some patients complain bitterly that, although they appear to sleep through the night, they waken 'unrefreshed' and tired, and must therefore sleep fitfully. This is sign of tension and reactive depression; if severe enough a MAOI should be prescribed.

The most commonly prescribed hypnotics today are nitrazepam and flurazepam, both benzodiazepines. Nitrazepam has a complex metabolism, and some of its metabolites are active. Flurazepam is metabolised rapidly, but its major metabolite has a very long half-life of 50 hours or more; accumulation may therefore occur, the patient continuing to feel sedated during the daytime. Flurazepam and nitrazepam, like other benzodiazepines, suppress stage 4 sleep. Flurazepam, unlike nitrazepam, does not suppress REM sleep and produce REM rebound. In small doses both drugs can of course be used as anxiolytics.

Chlormethiazole

A derivative of the thiazole part of thiamine, chlormethiazole is useful both as an anxiolytic and as a hypnotic, especially in elderly patients, in whom it rarely causes hypotension. But its main value is in the treatment of withdrawal states, particularly from alcohol.

It is a safe drug, but can cause dependence and should not generally be given for more than 4 weeks at a time. Up to 16 g of chlormethiazole a day may be needed in the treatment of delirium tremens. It can be given in the form of tablets, syrup, or by intravenous infusion. The drug's effects are potentiated by other tranquillisers and neuroleptics.

Side effects are few. The most common are sneezing, nasal irritation and conjunctival irritation.

Propranolol has been compared favourably to chlordiazepoxide in relieving anxiety. In fact the action of propranolol is mostly due to peripheral blockage of sympathetically mediated symptoms such as palpitations. The cutting short of such symptoms interrupts a feedback loop which would otherwise perpetuate the anxiety. Propranolol is indicated therefore when there are marked somatic symptoms; palpitations, diarrhoea, tremor. The dosage ranges from 30 to 240 mg a day.

The combination of a diazepine derivative with propranolol has advantages, combatting both the peripheral and central components of anxiety.

Propranolol in very high dosage has been advocated in the treatment of schizophrenia. Doses of up to 3 g a day have been used. This produces bradycardia, and sometimes severe hypotension and headache, but has little effect on psychotic symptoms. However, in doses of between 120 and 300 mg a day it does have a remarkably good effect in reducing, or stopping altogether, aggressive outburst in some psychotics and those with personality disorders.

FURTHER READING

Griffin, J.P., D'Arcy, P.F. 1979. *Manual of Adverse Drug Interactions*. Wright, Bristol.

Hollister, L.E. 1978. *Clinical Pharmacology of Psychotherapeutic Drugs*. Churchill Livingstone, Edinburgh.

Tyrer, P. 1973. Current status of monoamine oxidase inhibitions in psychiatry. *British Journal of Hospital Medicine* (June). 795–801.

Gershon, S., Shopsin, B. 1973. *Lithium; It's Role in Psychiatric Research and Treatment*. Plenum Press.

Schon, M., Amdisen, A., Baastrup, P.C. 1971. The practical management of lithium treatment. *British Journal of Hospital Medicine* (July). 53–59.

Brown, G.W., Birley, J.L.T., Wing, J.K. 1972. Influence of family life on the course of schizophrenia disorders. *British Journal of Psychiatry*. **121.** 245–258.

Lett, J.P. 1976. Assessment of drugs in schizophrenia. *British Journal of Clinical Pharmacology*. Suppl. 75–78.

Lett, J.P., Wing, J.K. 1971. Trial of maintenance therapy in schizophrenia. *British Medical Journal*. **3.** 599–604.

2

Electro-convulsion therapy

It was as long ago as 1798 that Weickhardt recommended the giving of camphor to the point of producing vertigo and epileptic fits for mental disorders, and other physicians followed his example. The treatment was revived in 1933 by Meduna, who, believing that schizophrenia and epilepsy were mutally antagonistic, gave intramuscular injections of 25 per cent solution of camphor in oil to schizophrenic patients. Camphor was replaced by better drugs, which could be given intravenously, or which would produce a fit more rapidly than by the older methods; cardiazol, triazol, picrotoxin. Finally, Cerletti and Bini in 1937 produced therapeutic fits by passing an electrical current between two electrodes placed on the forehead; a comparatively safe, convenient and painless method of convulsion therapy was thus made available.

Since that time the treatment has gone through more than one revolution. The objections of those who had thought that convulsion by chemical induction was brutal and inhumane were largely abandoned. Converts were rapidly made when it was discovered how effective the treatment was with sufferers from endogenous depression, how the risk of suicide was greatly reduced once effective treatment could be started, and how it was at last possible to treat many patients as outpatients. In the late 1940s muscle relaxants were introduced to lessen the risk of fractures, and then short-acting anaesthetics to mitigate the apprehension and anxiety of patients; thus 'modified' in the way still employed today, e.c.t. proved a powerful therapeutic tool.

Then came a period when the treatment was abused. In some hospitals it became a routine method of keeping patients, especially difficult schizophrenics, in a zombie-like state, easy to manage. Courses of twice-weekly e.c.t. were continued almost indefinitely, until some patients had had literally hundreds of treatments.

With the appearance of tranquillising drugs and antidepressants in the 1950s, this phase of overenthusiasm came to an end. There were even hopes that e.c.t. might be entirely replaced by drug therapy; but in fact no drug has yet appeared which equals modified e.c.t. for effectiveness, particularly speed of effect, in severe depressive illness.

Over the last 10 years e.c.t. has been subjected to much criticism, often ill-informed but occasionally justified. In the USA many psychiatrists are now reluctant to use e.c.t. at all, even in severe psychotic depression, for fear of litigation. The malpractice insurance premium is raised for the American physician who wishes to continue to prescribe e.c.t. As a result, psychiatrists have had to re-examine the possible risks, and the indications for its use. But acceptable controlled trials, where e.c.t. is compared with simulated e.c.t., both groups of patients receiving the same muscle relaxant and anaesthetic, are difficult to find, and ethically hard to justify in serious depression. Most studies confirm the effectiveness of e.c.t. compared to nonconvulsive treatment in affective psychoses. Today there can be few experienced psychiatrists who doubt the efficacy of e.c.t. in serious depression, and who have not at times seen a patient's life saved by such treatment.

Indications

Convulsive therapy was first used in the treatment of schizophrenia. However, it is in endogenous depressive illness that e.c.t. is so particularly effective. Over 70 per cent of patients with such a depression improve quickly with e.c.t. We have already discussed the difficulties of considering depressive illness as though it were a single entity. It is in serious endogenous depression that the results of convulsion therapy are so good. In the MRC trial (1965), comparing the effect of e.c.t. with imipramine, phenelzine and placebo, on 259 mental hospital patients with primary depressive illness severe enough to require admission, 71 per cent responded after 4 weeks, compared to 39 per cent given a placebo. At 6 months follow-up the percentage of patients treated with imipramine or e.c.t. alone who had recovered was the same. It is possible that imipramine, and presumably other antidepressants, have a cumulative antidepressant effect which, although slower, eventually catches up with that of e.c.t. Or, more likely, these figures reflect the spontaneous recovery rate of depression. In practice, of course, nowadays patients sufficiently depressed to need e.c.t. are treated concomitantly with antidepressant drugs.

Of all depressive syndromes those of later life react best to e.c.t. *Involutional melancholia* is a term that is tending to drop out of use, mainly because the grosser nihilistic delusions, agitation and hypochondria are uncommon symptoms today, probably because these patients receive effective treatment at a comparatively early stage in their illness. Unlike bipolar depression, involutional depressive symptoms often develop slowly and insidiously. At first the picture presented may be one that used to be called *neurasthenia*; the patient's interest and drive flags, everything becomes an effort, the world appears joyless, he retreats increasingly into himself, and hypochondriacal concern grows. Insomnia and depression of mood deepen, and without treatment there develops the full-blown picture of mixed agitation and retardation, with hypochondriacal preoccupation, ideas of guilt, and various delusions.

Recently Perris has attempted to differentiate unipolar from bipolar illness. His description of patients with unipolar illness fits the older ideas of involutional depression; patients tend to be asthenic, obsessional, tense, anxious and introverted (in contrast to the warmth and pyknic habitus of the manic depressive). Before the introduction of e.c.t. such agitated depressions had a poor prognosis, and drifted into chronicity in mental hospitals; indeed, it was these chronic involutional melancholics who responded so dramatically to the early use of e.c.t. in mental hospitals. But several studies have shown that involutional melancholia is not a strict entity, that it is made up of a number of genetically distinct syndromes and that involutional melancholia itself 'is only one element in a spectrum of depressive illnesses'.

Nonetheless e.c.t. has proved our most powerful weapon in the treatment of depressive illness in middle age. The prognosis with treatment is even more favourable now that e.c.t. can be supplemented with antidepressant drugs. Although there is a natural tendency to remit, depression seldom lifts spontaneously before 6 months, and often lasts 1 or 2 years. It may even extend into chronicity. The risk of death from exhaustion, intercurrent disease and suicide in the acute phase was, in the past, far from negligible.

High recovery rates with e.c.t. are only obtained in the central group of involutional depressives. Patients not of a previously rigid and obsessional personality, and those who have been of a markedly hysterical or anxious make-up do not do so well. Mood rhythm is important in selecting the most favourable patient. Early morning waking, and increased retardation and indecisiveness in the forenoon, are characteristic features of the depressions which respond favourably to e.c.t. Furthermore, there is a tendency to self-reproach, and a general lowering of vitality, shown in diminished libido.

Many patients in late middle life with symptoms of depression are of a different kind. Their illness is based on constitutional tendencies to anxiety. They have difficulty in getting to sleep, but do not usually waken early. They may begin the day well and feel at their worst in the evening. These patients are not such favourable subjects for e.c.t., and even when this treatment gives temporary help it often has to be supplemented by other methods. Depressed patients who suffer no disturbance of sleep are not, on the whole, helped by e.c.t.; many are made more anxious. In our experience also, patients whose libido is increased rather than diminished do not generally respond. But it is this group of 'neurotic' or 'atypical' depressives who do so well, provided they were previously of good personality, with the monoamine oxidase inhibitor group of antidepressant drugs.

Involutional depressions with the most favourable symptoms should be dealt with promptly. They can be readily treated in the psychiatric ward of a general hospital, and the risk of suicide is small if there is no delay. If the illness is recognised early, the patient can be treated as an outpatient, and the necessity for admission to hospital obviated. Time is important. As the illness advances the physical state of the patient deteriorates. The longer the patient is away from work, the more difficult it may become for him to go back. And finally, the sooner he begins treatment the more months of misery he and his family are spared. This of course does not mean that every middle-aged patient complaining of worry, insomnia and other depressive symptoms should be given e.c.t. at the first interview. Today, up to 60 per cent or more of patients with depression, who would have needed e.c.t. in the past, now respond to antidepressant drugs. It is perhaps a month before one can be sure whether the drugs are fully effective; and some patients may be too seriously depressed to wait this long. A prompt beginning should then be made with e.c.t., combined with a suitable antidepressant; the latter reduces the total number of treatments needed.

Depressions of the involutional type may occur very late in life, well into the period associated clinically with senile changes. If no organic basis in senile dementia or cerebral arteriosclerosis can be discovered, the outcome may be expected to be as favourable as in younger patients. Even when severe depressions are accompanied by the early stages of arteriosclerotic and senile dementia, they respond well to convulsion treatment; a high blood pressure or advanced age are certainly not contraindications to treatment which is justifiable on clinical grounds. The emotional lability of the organic patient must of course be distinguished from true depression.

Depression of mood, with marked paranoid features, may respond poorly to convulsion therapy, because the clinician has failed to notice its paraphrenic nature. It is important to recognise this group of patients, as their chances of recovery are prejudiced by incorrect treatment. A satisfactory remission can be obtained by combining the appropriate antidepressant and phenothiazine, together with e.c.t. if depression or paranoid delusions continue, but a maintenance dose of these drugs may be needed for some years to prevent relapse.

Manic depressive or bipolar syndromes

In depressions of earlier life, particularly before the age of 40, one should be rather more cautious over outcome. Perris has shown that bipolar illness starts 15 years or more sooner, on average, than unipolar depression, and is more likely to recur. The phasic changes of manic depression may be very troublesome to treat. It is not unusual for depression which has been relieved by convulsion therapy, to pass into hypomania which may prove even more difficult to manage, or depression may lift, but only temporarily, and return again every time e.c.t. is stopped. The swings of mood of manic depressives are largely endogenously determined, and dependent on biochemical changes at present beyond analysis and control. At times they seem to be more refractory to treatment than the involutional depressions, particularly in the early weeks, but spontaneous recovery may be awaited with much more certainty in manic depression.

The authors have seen many patients with recurrent depressive illnesses, who have been unsuccessfully handled. A patient may be treated on one occasion at the end of an attack with success, and is then told to present himself without delay for treatment when the next attack occurs. Several courses of e.c.t. are then given with only transient benefit; and when the patient eventually emerges of his own accord, at the end of his allotted span, he is labelled as having an hysterically motivated illness by the disappointed psychiatrist who has failed to recognise what he is dealing with.

With the introduction of antidepressant drugs and lithium the treatment of cyclothymic depressions has become considerably easier. Where medication is not sufficient by itself, and e.c.t. is subsequently combined with it, treatment has much more hope of success earlier in the attack than formerly. Provided the drug is continued, the improvement obtained with e.c.t. is likely to be stabilised, and the natural tendency to relapse held in check. The patient must be kept on an adequate dose of the antidepressant until the depressive cycle is obviously over. Relapse at any time, in spite of antidepressant drugs, calls for more e.c.t. If antidepressant drugs are stopped prematurely the handling of the case becomes muddled and difficult.

When we turn to consider the manic states, we find that convulsion therapy plays a much smaller part nowadays than it used to do. The first line of attack is with phenothiazines or haloperidol, backed up in many cases by lithium salts. The right dosage of one or other of these, or all in combination, usually obviates the need for e.c.t.

E.c.t., however, is still occasionally needed to control mania. Treatment needs to be given once or even twice a day, and the anaesthetic combined with intravenous haloperidol, 20 mg. Three or 4 days of convulsive treatment are usually enough to bring symptoms under control, after which drugs alone are sufficient.

Many states of acute excitement in young people, clinically resembling mania (and not drug induced), prove eventually to be schizophrenic; it is important to be on the alert for this possibility, so that appropriate treatment is not unnecessarily delayed.

Reactive depression

In reactive depressive states considerable expertise is called for therapeutically. Many people who, under environmental stress, become depressed have the rigid and obsessional temperament which one sees in the involutional depressive. Once driven into a state of depression by force of circumstances, the patient seems unable to find his way out. While first trying antidepressant drugs, the possibility of convulsion therapy should be borne in mind. If the environmental causes of depression are disposed of, but the patient still remains depressed, a few modified convulsions may be all that is required to break the vicious circle and start him on the road to recovery. It is in this group that early morning wakening and apprehension can be such useful pointers to success. When e.c.t. is given it is advisable to sedate the patient before treatment—sodium amylobarbitone 200 mg is more effective than diazepam in such cases—and to give 5 mg haloperidol or 10 mg diazepam with the anaesthetic. This lessens the anxiety which so often occurs in these patients after e.c.t., and may interfere with progress.

It is otherwise with reactive depression that occurs on the basis of an anxious temperament, and where the greatest mistakes are made. Here sleep may be normal, or there may be the typical initial insomnia seen in anxiety states. During the day mood fluctuates and shows no constant rhythm. Patients respond to changes in their environment and can be temporarily distracted from their woes by cheerful company. They have often been ill for a long time. E.c.t. is begun with mistaken enthusiasm, and continued even though the patient shrinks in fear from the treatment. Great harm can be done in this way, and the last state of the patient may be worse than the first. Fortunately, this group of reactive, or atypically depressed patients, who do so badly with e.c.t., do well with the MAOI group of antidepressants, combined when necessary with small doses of tranquillising drugs. Where clinical judgment fails, the results of one or two treatments often indicate the true nature of the illness. The depressed patient who is going to respond to e.c.t. often feels somewhat better after the first treatment for an hour or so, though depression then returns, and better for up to 24 hours after the third. The patient whose predominant symptoms are due to anxiety feels more tense after each treatment, (although the first e.c.t. may sometimes produce a dramatic transitory improvement).

Schizophrenia

Convulsion therapy was first used in the treatment of schizophrenia in the mistaken belief that epilepsy and schizophrenia were incompatible. On its own, it has never been highly regarded, and is certainly in no way comparable to the actions of the neuroleptics. Before their introduction, e.c.t. was considered to be inferior to insulin coma therapy. Both are probably nonspecific in their effect on schizophrenia.

Today the neuroleptics are without doubt first choice in the treatment of schizophrenia. In a previous edition of this book it was said that all recently ill schizophrenic patients should be given a neuroleptic drug, together with convulsion therapy, as soon as possible. There is indeed evidence to suggest that the action of a neuroleptic may be speeded up, and the amount of time a patient spends in hospital shortened, but this may not always be an advantage; when for instance there are strong emotional pressures at home, and time is needed to resolve them.

Our policy is to withhold e.c.t. initially, unless there is a strong depressive component, or confusion without organic cause. If the patient fails to show signs of improvement after a fortnight of adequate drug treatment, e.c.t. should be considered. Although trials have given inconclusive results, in our experience certain patients only begin to improve when e.c.t. is added to phenothiazine medication. Such patients tend to be older than average, of obsessional personality, and paranoid symptoms are usually evident. Whether e.c.t. actually enhances the antipsychotic action of the neuroleptic, lifts a masked depression which has been overlooked, or breaks up abnormal patterns of behaviour and thought, is unclear and is a fruitful field for research.

In schizo-affective disorders, when affective symptoms may be so prominent as to lead to a mistaken diagnosis of mania, e.c.t. is an invaluable adjunct to the neuroleptics. Disruptive behaviour ceases, frightening delusions vanish, the patient becomes responsive to staff and other patients, and is now able to benefit from supportive therapy. Catatonic stupor usually responds rapidly and dramatically to e.c.t. A treatment on two or three successive days may be all that is required. At times this can be lifesaving, for neuroleptics are often slow to produce any improvement. E.c.t. alone is inadvisable; the patient may swing from stupor to catatonic excitement unless adequate doses of chlorpromazine or haloperidol are given from the start.

Depression is present in many schizophrenic patients. In the early stages of the illness, before personality deterioration has occurred, depression is an understandable reaction to puzzling and frightening perceptual changes. For the most part, this depression lifts during the patient's stay in hospital. It is not advisable to give a patient antidepressant drugs in addition to neuroleptics immediately after admission. Side effects may be troublesome, and schizophrenic signs and symptoms enhanced. If depression is severe initially, then e.c.t. should be given rather than antidepressants. But when depression persists, or develops as schizophrenic symptoms disappear—and depressive symptoms occur in at least 50 per cent of schizophrenics treated with or maintained on neuroleptic drugs—an antidepressant drug can be added; in most cases there is then no need for e.c.t.

E.c.t. is of no value in simple or burnt out schizophrenia. Such patients show little affect and drive, and drift aimlessly from one day to the next. Regrettably we have no specific treatment at present which helps these unfortunate people.

Depersonalisation

Depersonalisation can occur in a variety of conditions; depression, anxiety and phobic anxiety states, schizophrenia, and some organic states. Among the latter we must include the injudicious or excessive use of e.c.t. Depersonalisation is a particular risk when e.c.t. is given to a very anxious and tense patient. It is for this reason, among others, that when e.c.t. has to be given to such a patient, we sedate him heavily 2 or 3 hours before treatment, and give a tranquillising drug intravenously with the anaesthetic; the patient then wakens some hours after e.c.t., relaxed and cheerful.

Depersonalisation is a common symptom of phobic anxiety states, particularly agoraphobia. Many patients respond excellently to a MAOI combined with a tranquilliser. Others respond to a tricyclic antidepressant, and a behavioural approach. Occasionally depersonalisation continues, when other symptoms of anxiety have vanished.

Roth's technique of intravenous thiopentone is sometimes successful, but a few patients have to endure years of discomfort. E.c.t. is generally contraindicated but when depersonalisation occurs as a symptom of agitated depression, especially the unipolar type, e.c.t. gives good results.

Hypochondriasis

Hypochondriasis is a preoccupation with a real or supposed physical or mental disorder, far out of proportion to the actual cause, if any, which exists; and which is not readily open to explanation and persuasion. Hypochondriasis develops in the setting of depression, anxiety and phobic anxiety, in schizophrenia, where it sometimes takes bizarre forms, obsessional states, and in organic states, particularly of old age. When hypochondriacal concern appears after the onset of depression, antidepressant treatment, including e.c.t., is likely to remove it, along with other depressive symptoms. But when the patient has always been of an introspective, hypochondriacal nature, when depression is dominated by hypochondriacal concern, then antidepressant treatment, while improving other symptoms of depression, is unlikely completely to remove hypochondriasis. Several studies have indicated that the response of depressed patients to e.c.t., in the presence of hypochondriasis, is poor. Clearly there is no clinical justification for giving large numbers of e.c.t. to such patients.

There is disagreement as to whether hypochondriasis can exist in its own right, in a primary or essential form. Certainly we see patients who have been hypochondriacal for many years, often from their late teens or early twenties. Hypochondriasis seems to start during a time of anxiety or reactive depression, often following clumsy handling or advice by a doctor, and then becomes a fixture. The patient's emotional needs and problems come to be expressed increasingly in terms of hypochondriacal concern. It is often impossible to convince him that he is healthy, in spite of inclusive tests and examinations. Anxiety is often present, and the condition runs a phasic course. Male patients usually stick to one organ symptom; the heart, the gastrointestinal system, the head. Women, on the other hand, can present in a more protean way, switching from one system to another. The best known description of such patients is Briquet's syndrome; women who, before the age of 35, have attended doctors with at least 25 symptoms in 9 out of 10 body systems. They are regarded by researchers as hysterics. E.c.t. does little good here.

Anxiety neurosis

The use of convulsions in chronic anxiety neurosis is, as a rule, to be avoided. Where the neurosis is of recent origin and has clear cut precipitants, readjustment of the patient's environment, psychotherapy, and use of sedatives and antidepressants, are much more likely to be of service. Where the neurosis is of long-standing and largely constitutional, no benefit from e.c.t. can be expected. Most patients with the label 'anxiety neurosis' who benefit from this treatment have been wrongly diagnosed and are in fact suffering from depression, with agitation to the fore. If a patient with an excellent personality and no past neurotic history suddenly, and for the first time between the ages of 30 and 55, presents with what seems to be a severe anxiety state, an underlying depression should always be suspected. It is likely to respond to e.c.t. and antidepressants.

Hysteria

Conversion hysteria may be cleared by a single convulsion, as by any other dramatic method of treatment; but less drastic methods are more appropriate. Not infrequently, depressed patients exhibit hysterical symptoms as a reaction to the difficulties caused by their illness. When depression clears, hysterical symptoms go with them. Especially in the middle-aged woman, a hysterical superstructure may almost completely mask the underlying depression. We have met a number of patients, on the surface seemingly chronic neurotics, anxious and with a multitude of hypochondriacal symptoms, but who coped well with their lives before the illness began. These patients improved when given e.c.t. and antidepressants. In some cases the illness was of long duration; what probably started as a depressive state took on hysterical features, which masked the depression and came to dominate the patient's behaviour and the attitudes of people close to her.

Hysterical and anxious patients are more prone than most to develop memory disturbances after e.c.t., and then to make them the subject of bitter complaint. If e.c.t. has to be given, side effects should be guarded against by heavy sedation before treatment, and the use of intravenous tranquillisers with, or immediately after the anaesthetic. The number of e.c.t. in such cases rarely need exceed three or four.

Obsessional neurosis

Similar principles hold for obsessional neuroses. Convulsion therapy does not help patients with primary obsessive compulsive illness. Persistent attempts to create effects which are not obtainable are only likely to add to the patient's difficulties. Some become obsessed by disturbance of memory. Others develop depersonalisation.

It has already been pointed out that the obsessional personality is particularly liable to severe depression, which may persist for an undue length of time. For such patients e.c.t. offers considerable hope. It is not unusual to find a mixture of obsessional and phobic symptoms in a depressive psychosis, particularly of later life. A depressed woman may, for instance, complain that she is haunted by a fear that she may destroy her children; every time she goes to the knife box she is seized afresh with the idea. Patients such as this are very suitable for treatment by convulsion, but they can hardly be called obsessionals in the strict sense. A number of obsessional patients, dominated by depression and tension, are now helped by antidepressants, which often avoids the need for e.c.t.

Other conditions

Up to recent times some psychiatrists appeared to believe that they needed only two weapons in their armoury; psychotherapy and the electric shock box, one sure where the other failed. Thus the literature records the use of e.c.t. in almost every imaginable psychiatric condition, from GPI to a stammer. It is always possible to produce change of a kind by e.c.t. But if the appropriate indications are absent the patient gains nothing thereby, for symptoms usually quickly return, sometimes worse than before. There are, however, some special cases in which even temporary relief is of vital consequence, i.e. when the symptom is itself of short duration, but while it lasts constitutes a serious danger. We have already mentioned the use of e.c.t as an emergency treatment of life-threatening behaviour in schizophrenia and depressive stupor. Rarely e.c.t. may be needed in anorexia nervosa; usually with a chronic patient who seems resolved on starving herself to death. E.c.t. is then used to break the patient's resistance to eating. It is distasteful, but preferable to forcible tube feeding. Of 400 patients seen over the past 10 years, we have had to give e.c.t. on one occasion only (see p. 121).

E.c.t. can prove valuable when a depressive illness appears in disguise. We have, for instance, seen hypochondriacal states, and conditions where the dominant symptom is pain, clear up with e.c.t. after many years duration. In all these patients, the underlying depression had previously been overlooked, although to the wary there were unmistakeable marks of an affective change.

It must not be argued, from this narrowly limited group, that it is justifiable to treat psychosomatic states of all kinds with e.c.t. Most such conditions, when they are based on emotional change, can be traced to long continuing anxiety and tension. They are often made worse by e.c.t., seldom benefited.

Risks and contraindications

It can hardly be sufficiently emphasised that convulsion therapy is a surgical treatment in psychiatry, and the general rules governing the admissibility of surgical intervention apply. While the operation should not be unnecessarily delayed, it should not be undertaken in a light-hearted spirit, and should never be employed as a mere placebo. When e.c.t. is decided on, the patient should be medically examined to exclude possible dangers, the position should be explained both to him and his relatives, and the permission of both obtained. Finally, when the treatment is eventually carried out, every effort should be used to minimise special risks.

The risk of death with convulsion therapy is very small. Studies suggest a mortality of around 0·0036 per cent; that is 3 to 4 deaths per 100 000 treatments. Compare this risk with the mortality of untreated depression before the advent of e.c.t., around 15 per cent. Ultimately, it is the responsibility of the psychiatrist to decide on a patient's fitness for treatment, and whether the probable benefits of e.c.t. outweigh the possible risks. If he has any doubts about the physical state of the patient he should initiate appropriate investigations; chest X-ray, e.c.g. and so on, and ask the advice of a physician.

It must be emphasised again that e.c.t. is an extremely safe treatment when given by *experienced medical* personnel. In the rare event of death—the danger period is after e.c.t., during the recovery stage—this is nearly always due to cardiovascular complications, usually cardiac arrhythmias. Obviously the risk is greater the more diseased the heart. A recent myocardial infarct is a strong contraindication to e.c.t. Even with a well modified convulsion there is a short-lived but large rise of blood pressure. A history of a past cerebrovascular accident calls for careful consideration. Serious chest disease and heart failure may cause worry to the anaesthetist; this can only be alleviated by close understanding and co-operation between him and the psychiatrist. The presence of a pacemaker is generally no contraindication to e.c.t.; but it is sensible to discuss the question of treatment fully with the patient's cardiologist. Age is no contraindication to e.c.t., nor is a mild degree of dementia alongside severe depression.

There are in fact few serious complications to e.c.t., provided patients are carefully selected, treatment is carried out correctly and not prolonged unnecessarily, and steps are taken to reduce severe anxiety, both before and after convulsion.

Ideally, a patient should be allowed to waken naturally. With very anxious patients we like to give intravenous haloperidol 5 mg, or diazepam 10 mg, at the time of the anaesthetic, or immediately after the fit (diazepam does not usually prevent the convulsion, but if it appears to do so haloperidol is given instead). Sleep may be prolonged by this medication for anything up to 2 or 3 hours, and the patient wakens relaxed and without the headache and agitation that occasionally develop in very tense patients. However, we recognise that this is not always possible.

Some degree of confusion is seen in about 10 per cent of patients when they first awaken. It is more likely to occur in older patients, and confusion that is marked and prolonged beyond say 15 minutes should call for careful reassessment of the patient, and consideration as to whether e.c.t. should continue. Headache is troublesome in about 15 per cent of patients, but wears off after an hour or so, helped if necessary by an analgesic. Other complaints, such as muscle stiffness, and drowsiness, are due more to the muscle relaxant and anaesthetic than to the fit itself. Fractures were not uncommon before the use of muscle relaxants, but are now very unusual.

Memory disturbance, particularly for verbal memory, is greater following bilateral than unilateral e.c.t. It is also more common in patients who fail to respond well to e.c.t.; this is not necessarily because they have more treatments, but may well indicate that patients have not been wisely selected. Patients with much anxiety often complain that they cannot recall past events, are unable to remember the names of acquaintances, and say that learning has become harder. These complaints are of course subjective, and are difficult to confirm. They sometimes become the centre of a patient's symptomatology.

It is important to bear in mind that depression itself impairs memory, by lessening attention and concentration, and so reducing learning ability. Immediately after a fit there is a mild degree of retrograde amnesia, and learning is transiently impaired. Memory disturbance increases with the number of treatments given, and with the amount of electricity passed. Modern techniques aim to restrict the current to a minimum necessary to produce a fit.

There is no good evidence that e.c.t. causes brain damage. Nor is there any objective evidence of permanent memory impairment. However, some patients (virtually restricted to those who are not helped by e.c.t.) continue to complain of poor memory for many years after a course of treatment. As we have said, however, memory disturbance is a common symptom in affective disorders.

A vexatious complication of e.c.t. is translation of depression into mania or hypomania. A mild degree of euphoria is common in all types of depression after quick resolution, but this soon settles and creates no problems. Only in manic depressive patients is mania liable to replace depression and require treatment. Particularly when the illness is recognised to be a bipolar affective condition, monitoring the progress after each treatment should give adequate warning, allowing e.c.t. to be stopped in time, and precautions taken. Schizo-affective disorders and catatonic stupor may also be switched rapidly into states of excitement by e.c.t., unless the psychiatrist is constantly alert to be possibility. We cannot emphasise enough that e.c.t. must go hand in hand with ongoing assessment of the patient, not as a set course of treatments.

Number of treatments

E.c.t. is highly effective in endogenous depression, but in the past, before antidepressant drugs became available, at least 25 per cent of patients relapsed and needed further e.c.t. The average number of treatments (bilateral e.c.t.) was 8. In order to minimise the risk of relapse it was common practice to give two extra e.c.t. after apparent recovery. Today, antidepressant drugs are almost invariably given with e.c.t. Not only do they lessen the possibility of relapse (most of our patients now need between 4 and 6 unilateral e.c.t.), but they reduce the number of e.c.t. needed. Any of the antidepressant drugs in current use can be given concomitantly, including the MAOI. There are no additional complications and risks, apart from increased postural hypotension during the post- e.c.t. recovery stage.

Neuroleptics and tranquillisers may also be given safely with e.c.t. Reserpine is the only drug that is contraindicated with e.c.t.

Unilateral or bilateral e.c.t.

It is now clear that unilateral e.c.t., where the current is applied only to the nondominant hemisphere, produces less memory disturbance than bilateral e.c.t., or when the current is administered to the dominant side. However, it is also apparent that unilateral is not as effective as bilateral e.c.t. in severe depression. More treatments are then required, and the patient has to wait longer for depression to lift; the ever attendant risk of suicide is therefore prolonged. Our own practice is to give e.c.t. unilaterally to most patients, except when depression is severe and suicide is a risk; then we invariably give bilateral e.c.t.

It is sometimes difficult to discover the dominant hemisphere. Even in patients who seem to be strongly right-handed a 10 per cent error exists. Patients should be asked not only which hand they preferentially use, but whether this has always been so. It may also be helpful to inquire about the dominant foot and eye.

Administration of e.c.t., both inpatient and outpatient

E.c.t. should be administered in a special room. It should, ideally, have two doors, one by which to enter and another leading into a recovery room, so that the waiting patient does not hear or see the treated patient; which can be an upsetting experience.

In the e.c.t. room are the anaesthetist, the psychiatrist and nursing staff. The patient may need to be reassured, not only while waiting but also as he enters the room. The anaesthetist will want to check that the patient has had nothing to eat or drink during the previous 5 hours. A patient who is unduly anxious can be calmed by means of a tranquilliser, given 1 to 2 hours before treatment. Dentures are usually taken out, and shoes removed for we observe the toes for the jerks that indicate a fit.

The anaesthetist should be able easily to see the results of the physical examination and investigations in the patient's notes. Included with the notes is the e.c.t. form containing the patient's written consent. It is helpful, from the point of view of subsequent treatments, for this form to include salient points from the physical examination, the patient's current drugs, and a record of previous e.c.t.s, with doses of anaesthetic, muscle relaxant and atropine given, the intensity of the last convulsion, and any complications. In addition, a book should be provided in which the anaesthetist and psychiatrist record details of each e.c.t. given.

The dangers of e.c.t. are few, as we have emphasised, but emergency equipment should be present in the e.c.t. room. This should include a sucker, endo-tracheal tubes, stimulant drugs, reserves of oxygen, telephone, and ideally, a defibrillator.

Anaesthetic induction

Atropine 0·6 to 2 mg is given first, preferably intravenously. This not only dries up secretions but lessens the risk of arrhythmias and of vagal overstimulation.

The anaesthetic. Thiopentone is often preferred to methohexitone because of its longer action, allowing the patient to sleep later, and thereby to be more relaxed on waking. Patients should, if possible, be allowed to waken naturally, rather than be roused by a nurse, but space does not always permit this.

The muscle relaxant. A muscle relaxant such as succinylcholine (Scoline), or suxemethonium (Brevedil-E), is given immediately after the anaesthetic. The dosage varies, depending on a patient's size and medical condition. It is important that the dose should not be so large that the physical convulsion is no longer apparent.

There is good evidence that the efficacy of e.c.t. is dependent on the seizure; clinical experience suggests that a subconvulsion or non-generalized seizure is not only therapeutically less effective, but may be positively harmful. It is therefore standard practice to ensure that a bilateral convulsion occurs with both bilateral and unilateral e.c.t.

Rarely a patient is deficient in pseudo-cholinesterase, the enzyme concerned with metabolising the muscle relaxant. The paralysing effect of the drug is then prolonged, and the return of natural respiration may be delayed, sometimes for several hours.

The patient is now oxygenated. There is evidence that this procedure lessens possible memory disturbances after e.c.t. A mouth gag is inserted.

The convulsion. There is a variety of apparatus for giving e.c.t. One with a choice of waveforms, and with automatic timing, is preferable to one without such calibrations, since this allows the current to be kept at the minimum needed to produce a convulsion. The order of current passed is 25 to 40 joules. If a convulsion does not occur the procedure should be repeated, up to three times, until convulsion occurs. A subconvulsion is liable to produce anxiety, headache and other side effects. It is claimed that, by positioning electrodes over the frontal or occipital areas instead of the fronto-temporal areas generally used, memory disturbance is lessened. There is no incontrovertible evidence that this is so. For unilateral e.c.t. the electrodes are usually placed over the parietal and frontal regions of the non-dominant side.

Recovery. After the convulsion the patient is oxygenated, with an airway *in situ*, and remains in the e.c.t. room under the care of the anaesthetist until respiration returns and consciousness is regained. Close nursing observation is needed at this time, because this is when a patient may choke, stop breathing, or suffer cardiac arrest.

He is then moved out to the recovery room, where a qualified nurse should be in attendance. Reassurance and explanation when the patient comes round are important and help to lessen agitation. Although each patient has treatment alone he will, because of lack of space, usually recover in the company of others. Once he has woken completely and is orientated, he is helped from the recovery room to a comfortable chair in the anteroom, or back to his bed in the ward, where he is given tea and sandwiches and usually rests for an hour or so. An analgesic may be helpful if headache is pronounced or prolonged.

Frequency of e.c.t. Daily or twice daily convulsions, although occasionally still used in otherwise uncontrollable mania, do not increase the rate of recovery from depression. Most psychiatrists give e.c.t. twice a week, and this is our practice. Spacing of e.c.t. closer than 48-hour intervals probably increases memory disturbance with little or no additional therapeutic gain.

Medico-legal

Patients should always, if possible, give written consent for a course of e.c.t. If a patient is informal and unwilling, e.c.t. cannot be given. Problems only arise if a patient is compulsorily detained and is unwilling, or unable for whatever reason, to agree to treatment, and yet e.c.t. is thought to be essential. Present legal advice is that if e.c.t. is to be given, such a patient should be detained under Section 26 rather than Section 25 of the Mental Health Act (1959). Except in an emergency, when the consultant can act on his own initiative, two consultant opinions on the need for e.c.t. should be obtained. It is also advisable to discuss the matter with the patient's nearest relative and obtain his or her written agreement.

FURTHER READING

Cronholm, B., Ottosson, J.O. 1960. Experimental studies of the therapeutic action of ECT in endogenous depression. *Acta Psychiatrica Scandinavica,* Suppl. 145. **35**. 69.

Cronin, D. et al. 1970. Unilateral and bilateral ECT; a study of memory disturbance and relief from depression. *J. Neurology, Neurosurgery, and Psychiatry*. **33**. 705.

Fink, M. 1977. Myths of shock therapy. *Amer. J. Psychiatry.* **134**. 991.

Gomez, J., Dally, P. 1975. ECT and i.v. sedation. *Brit. J. Psychiatry.* **127**. 604.

Greenblatt, M., Grosser, G.H., Wechsler, H. 1964. Differential response of hospitalised depressed patients to somatic therapy. *Amer. J. Psychiatry.* **120**. 935.

Medical Research Council, 1965. Clinical trial of the treatment of depressive illness. *Brit. Med. J.* **1**. 881.

Perris, C. 1966. A study of bipolar and unipolar depressive psychoses. *Acta Psychiatrica Scandinavica*. Suppl. 194.

The Royal College of Psychiatrists. 1977. Memorandum on the use of electroconvulsive therapy. *Brit. J. Psychiatry.* **131**. 261.

3

Psychosurgery

Understandably, the effectiveness and ethics of psychosurgery have been increasingly questioned in recent years. Many patients in the past—and particularly in the immediate post-war years—were operated on without fully understanding the nature of the operation, and sometimes without being capable of such understanding. Emotional reactions inevitably coloured the question of whether or not to proceed to prefrontal leucotomy, not only in the patient but in his relatives and doctors. These were heightened by the fact that leucotomy was, and frequently still is, seen as a 'last resort', a final, desperate, irreversible step, all other treatments having failed.

Discussion of the procedures available, their indications and contra-indications, their unwanted as well as their desirable effects, has all too often been more journalistic than scientific. Reviews can sometimes resemble missionary tracts, political pamphlets or lampoons. This is largely because there have been no satisfactory controlled trials of psychosurgical procedures, for obvious reasons.

There are important legal and ethical issues about, for example, what constitutes informed consent (particularly poignant in the subnormal and in children), and surrounding the surgical damage of human brains that are intact though, at some level, dysfunctional. Psychosurgery, on this view, would be countenanced if it were done for pyschiatric illness but not solely to change behaviour. Unfortunately, there is no universal agreement as to what is, or is not, psychiatric illness.

The debate about psychosurgery revolves around its objectives and its means. Its objectives are to improve the quality of the patient's life, and enable him to develop a more satisfactory and satisfying relationship with his fellows. The means are the procedures discussed in this chapter. The fact that they have sometimes been used on non-consenting, ill-informed persons is a matter for shame, but it should not detract from consideration of their proper application. Abuse does not negate use; a razor can slit a throat but most people find it useful for shaving.

The history of psychosurgical procedures is well known, and is reviewed in several other places. For the purposes of this book, it need only be said that there has been a convergence of evidence from patients who have suffered brain injury, from neurophysiological experimentation on primates, and from the results of the several psychosurgical procedures that have been employed since leucotomy was introduced in the 1930s. This evidence strongly suggests that disconnection of the association tracts between the frontal lobe cortex and limbic lobe results in reduction of unwanted emotions, and their autonomic and motor accompaniments.

Public debate on psychosurgery in the United States led to the setting up of the National Commission for the Protection of Human Subjects from Biomedical and Behavioural Research. In 1977 it produced its findings. Medically qualified members were in a minority. It seems to have surprised itself in finding a distinct but limited usefulness for psychosurgery, with small 'cost' from the brain tissue destruction.

Older 'free hand' operations, to disconnect the frontal lobe from the limbic lobe, have now been superseded by modern stereotactic operations. Results of these earlier procedures can be found in older reviews. Some of them are summarised in Table 3.1. It will be noted that among 10 365 standard prefrontal leucotomies done in Britain in the 10 years after 1942, there was a *good response* among 50 per cent of the depressives and 18 per cent of the schizophrenics. Bridges has argued that this latter low figure of 'good response' should be judged against the then prevailing poor outcome of chronic schizophrenia, in the period

Table 3.1 Approximate comparisons of the results and side effects of various psychosurgical operations (From Bridges, P.K. In *A Contemporary View of Psychosurgery*. Ed. Gaind, R., Hudson, B. Current Themes in Psychiatry – 1, 1978. McMillan, London)

	Standard prefrontal (Tooth and Newton, 1961)	Bimedial (Birley, 1964)	Orbital undercut (Sykes and Tredgold, 1964)
n =	10365	92	350
Good response for:			
Depression	50%	50%	69%
Anxiety	—	—	44%
Obsessional neurosis	—	75%	30%
Schizophrenia	18%	—	31%[d]
Effects on the personality (see notes)	3.1%[a]	6.9%[c]	5%[e]
Fits	1.3%[b]	1%	16%[f]
Deaths	0.3%	0	1.5%

a Severe enough to prevent discharge.
b Persisting at time of review.
c 'Quite severe changes'.
d 4 of 13.
e 'Incapacity produced by multiple behaviour changes'.
f One or more fits.

before the advent of phenothiazines.

Modern stereotactic procedures produce lesions only millimetres wide, which are sited after electrical stimulation has allowed for accurate placement. The physician wanting to help his patient give informed consent will need to know the procedures available, the indications and contraindications so far recognised, the probable outcome, and the hazards involved; in fact, the cost-benefit.

Conditions treated psychosurgically

It is in mood disorders that the best results from psychosurgery have been obtained. The precise diagnosis is less important than the presence of certain key symptoms of disabling severity. These are depression, anxiety, and obsession/compulsion, which are prolonged and intractable. *Prolonged* means, in practice, of several years' duration, though a more rapid recourse to psychosurgery is urged by some of its proponents. *Intractable* implies that no other treatment, properly and persistently applied, has relieved the disorder, or reduced the frequency and severity of recurring illness. *Disabling* describes an inability to sustain work and a reasonably normal social life.

Pain, unrelieved by other means, sometimes comes to psychosurgery. In some patients the operation is followed by dramatic and immediate relief; in others, the severity of the pain, according to the patient, is unaffected but the unpleasant affect is now detached from the experience, which becomes more bearable.

More controversial is the use of psychosurgery in obesity, violence, sexual deviation and childhood hyperactivity. In Britain, psychosurgical teams insist on the informed consent of patients when they are voluntary patients, free to decide whether or not to have surgery. Psychosurgery carried out on the subnormal, and on chronic psychotic patients detained under the 1959 Mental Health Act, carries serious doubts about the nature of the consent obtained.

Neuronal pathways

The neuronal pathways of current psychosurgical interest are the frontal lobe cortex, dorsal and orbital, and its white matter connections, especially through its lower medial quadrant to and from the limbic lobe. The latter comprises cortex and association tracts, linking nuclear masses concerned with emotional experience and its autonomic accompaniment. Its main constituents are: the cingulate gyrus and bundle, hippocampus, amygdala, hypothalamus, mamillary bodies, fornix and thalamus. The linkages are circuit-like and are depicted in Figures 3.1 and 3.2.

The major fronto-limbic connection traverses the lower medial quadrant of the frontal lobe, carrying receptor fibres to, and effector

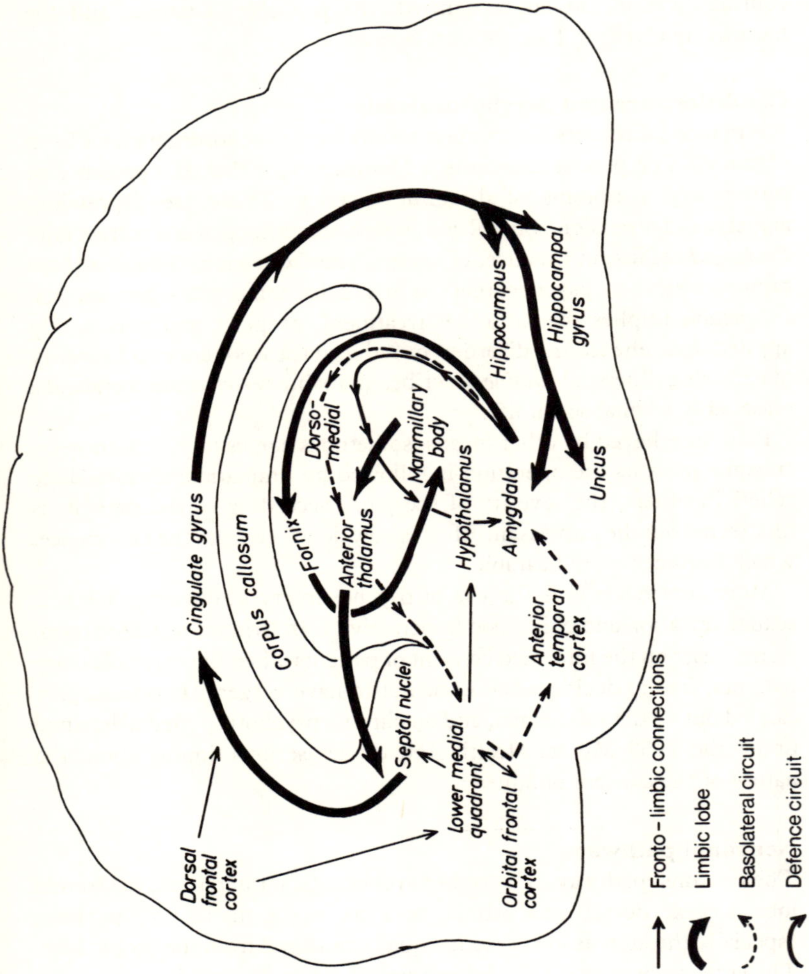

Fig. 3.1 The limbic lobe and its connections relevant to psychosurgery

fibres from the frontal cortex, to the nuclei of the septum and the hypothalamus. Additionally, there is a direct association tract from the dorsal frontal cortex, thence to the amygdala, on to the dorsal medial nuclei of the thalamus, and back to the orbital cortex.

Electrical stimulation of its various nuclei and tracts gives rise in animals to changes in heart rate, blood pressure, respiration and the supply of blood to muscles, as well as in aggressive, appetitive and sexual behaviour. In conscious man, stimulation of the area evokes similar autonomic changes, and the experience of anxiety and/or aggressive feelings.

The Papez circuit runs from the cingulate gyrus and its bundle to the hippocampus, thence through the fornix to the mamillary bodies and, by way of the anterior nuclei of the thalamus, back to the cingulum. A smaller 'defence circuit' links hypothalamus with amygdala. Electrical stimulation of the area suggests that it is intimately involved in the preparation for 'flight or fight'.

Lewin has postulated that the prolonged unwanted emotional states, which psychosurgery seeks to treat, are due to 'reverberating circuits'; an almost perpetual motion of neuronal discharges around the fronto-limbic connections, the Papez, and 'defence' circuits.

With the failure of all other treatments (environmental manipulation,

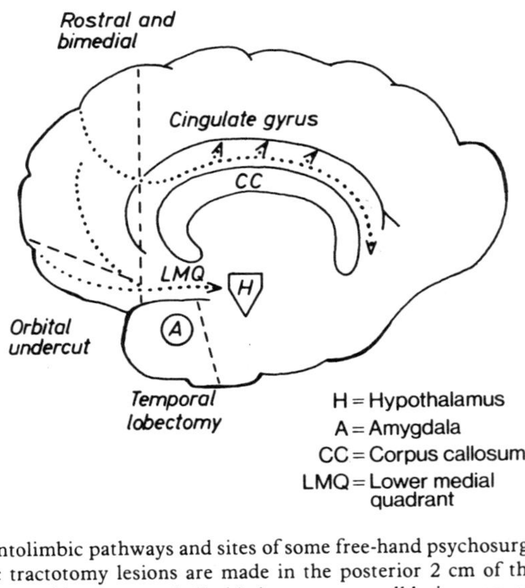

Fig. 3.2 Frontolimbic pathways and sites of some free-hand psychosurgical procedures. In stereotactic tractotomy lesions are made in the posterior 2 cm of the orbital undercutting incision, and in stereotactic limbic leucotomy small lesions are made in the lower medial quadrant (LMQ) of the frontal lobe and in the cingulum bundle (dotted) in the cingulate gyrus. The amygdala (A) and hypothalamus (H) are target sites for operations on the defence reaction circuit for uncontrollable violence associated with epilepsy (Reproduced from 1976. *Brit. J. Hosp. Med.* August.)

psychotherapy, both interpretive and behavioural, and all appropriate physical treatment), psychosurgery aims to interrupt these circuits. The lesions produced are small nowadays, in terms of millimetres, large in relation to the number of neuronal fibres destroyed.

Contraindications to psychosurgery

Leucotomy has nothing to offer patients with lifelong inadequate personalities; who have little persistence, repeatedly fail to cope with their responsibilities, flit from job to job, and constantly blame everyone but themselves for their misfortunes. Marked psychopathic personality traits and antisocial features are also strong contraindications; serious alcohol or drug abuse, persistent and uncontrollable violence, and socially unacceptable sexual deviations, are predictors of poor response to the prefrontal leucotomies. Age is no contraindication. Indeed, the later the onset of an illness the better, but the presence of dementia obviously militates against success.

Any tendency to bleed, and signs of hypertension and arteriosclerosis, are absolute contraindications to operate.

Commoner present day procedures

1. *Stereotactic tractotomy*

In this operation the association fibres in the ventromedial quadrant beneath the caudate nuclei of both frontal lobes are interrupted stereotactically. The aim is to disconnect the frontal lobe cortex from the limbic circuits. One series of more than 800 patients has been treated in this way, using Yttrium (Y^{90}) in ceramic rods. The lesions are about 25 mm by 15 mm by 5 mm. (The destruction of association tracts in other operations and centres has been achieved by cold, heat, or radiofrequency, as well as by division.)

A first series of 210 patients was reported to show a good response in 56 per cent of those who were operated on for depression; 40 per cent of those with anxiety; and 50 per cent of those with obsessions/compulsions. A second series of 208 patients reported a good response in 68 per cent, 63 per cent and 50 per cent respectively of those conditions. Fits occurred in 1 to 2 per cent. One death only resulted from the operation in the entire series of over 800. In the later series no significant adverse personality changes were noted. The results are summarised in Table 3.2.

2. *Limbic leucotomy*

Here, lesions of about 8 mm diameter are stereotactically induced by cryo-coagulation in the ventro-medial white matter of the frontal lobe, close to the site selected in sub-caudate tractotomy.

Table 3.2 Approximate comparisons of the results and side effects of various psychosurgical operations (From Bridges, P.K. In *A Contemporary View of Psychosurgery*. Ed. Gaind, R., Hudson, B. Current Themes in Psychiatry – 1, 1978, McMillan, London)

	Stereotactic tractotomy (Ström-Olsen and Carlisle, 1971)	Stereotactic tractotomy (Göktepe et al, 1975)	Limbic leucotomy (Mitchell-Heggs et, al, 1976)
n =	210	208	66
Good response for:			
Depression	56%	68%	56% [d]
Anxiety	41%	63%	27% [d]
Obsessional neurosis	50%	50%	67% [d]
Schizophrenia	0	0	57%[e]
Effects on the personality (see notes)	2·6%[a]	7%[b]	
Fits	1%	2%	
Deaths	0	one patient[c]	

a 'Moderate and lasting sequelae'.
b 'Not socially disabling'.
c One patient in the whole series of over 800 operations so far carried out.
d Improvement ratings I and II only, to make for comparison with other reports (Published as I, II and III)
e 4 of 7.

Increased heart rate, decreased frequency and amplitude of respiration, and increased forearm blood flow following electrical stimulation, confirm the precise siting of the probe in the anaesthetised patient before the lesion is made. Two additional lesions are sited in each anterior cingulate gyrus. Where marked anxiety and tension dominate the clinical picture, other lesions are made in the genu of the corpus callosum.

There are different views as to whether these additional cingulum and corpus callosum lesions add to a favourable outcome. A controlled study was planned by the Royal College of Psychiatrists to compare the two procedures, but difficulties with factions opposed to psychosurgery have regrettably halted the project.

Clinical ratings, psychological and physiological assessments before, at 6 weeks and 20 months after stereotactic limbic leucotomy, have been reported. At 20 months 63 per cent of patients with anxiety states, 61 per cent of those with depression and 84 per cent of obsessive compulsive neurotics were improved in some degree. Against that, 37 per cent, 39 per cent and 16 per cent of the same categories were unchanged or worse. These global clinical ratings are summarised in Table 3.3.

The Wechsler Adult Intelligence Scale (WAIS) scores actually improved after operation, though the authors attribute this in part to the effect of practice. Symptom-scores significantly fell as a whole for the group and there were significant improvements in some, though not all, of the basal and stress related physiological measurements.

Table 3.3 Clinical ratings 6 weeks and 20 months after limbic leucotomy (n = 148) (From Anxiety and Emotions; physiological basis and treatment by Desmond Kelly; Charles C. Thomas, 1980)

	6 weeks							20 months					
	N	I	II	III	IV	V	% of total improved	I	II	III	IV	V	% of total improved
Obsessional neurosis	49	2	22	14	11	0	78	7	23	11	5	3	84
Chronic anxiety	27	0	10	8	8	1	67	3	5	9	8	2	63
Depression	36	5	12	9	10	0	72	7	7	8	11	3	61
Schizophrenia	19	0	4	7	7	1	58	0	6	6	5	2	63
Other:													
Personality disorder	7	0	0	1	6	0		0	3	2	2	0	
Anorexia nervosa	5	0	0	3	2	0		1	0	0	3	1	
Depersonalization	1	0	0	0	0	1		0	0	0	0	1	
Intractable pain	1	0	1	0	0	0		0	0	1	0	0	
Dementia (depression)	1	0	0	0	1	0		0	0	0	0	1	
Paranoia	1	0	0	1	0	0		0	0	0	1	0	
Palilalia (Parkinsonism)	1	0	0	0	1	0		0	0	0	1	0	
							35						41
Total	148	7	49	43	46	3	67	18	44	37	36	13	67

I: Symptom-free IV: Not improved
II: Much improved V: Worse
III: Improved

Nineteen schizophrenic patients were operated on. None was symptom-free at 20 months but 12 were partially improved. Five were unchanged and two were worse. The authors argue that in spite of previous poor results in this condition, consideration of psychosurgery should not necessarily be ruled out.

3. *Anterior cingulotomy*

This procedure, besides being used as an alternative to those described above, has also been used for the relief of intractable pain. Less controversial measures, like posterior rhizotomy and chordotomy, may already have been unsuccessfully carried out. Small lesions are sited some 2·5 cm in front of the anterior horn of the lateral ventricles, 13 to 15 mm from the midline. Pain due to metastatic disease can sometimes be relieved, but only temporarily; some 3 to 6 months later it is liable to recur. It seems that new neuronal pathways are established, circumventing the surgical disconnection. No comparable phenomenon has been as sharply described following psychosurgical treatment of depression, anxiety and obsession compulsions.

Intractable pain has also been treated by stereotactic limbic leucotomy and subcaudate tractotomy. While relief of pain often follows immediately after surgery, improvement in mood disorders develops more slowly, over the weeks and months after operation. The reasons for these dissimilarities are obscure.

4. *Multifocal leuco-coagulation*

From this last observation, one neurological team implanted several gold electrodes and produced serial small coagulations over 6 months after the implantation, but infection along the tracks, from scalp to electrode, proved troublesome and this procedure has not been widely practised.

More rarely, lesions have been made in the hypothalamus in the treatment of obesity, and to diminish the drive of sexual deviants.

5. *Temporal lobectomy*

The results of temporal lobectomy in drug-resistant epilepsy originating from that lobe are good. More than half the patients cease to fit after the operation, and associated psychotic states and aggressive outbursts also often improve. The lesion usually found at operation, and with the best outlook, is mesial temporal sclerosis, involving the uncus, amygdala and hippocampus. Less often present, and less responsive to operation, are hamartomas, scars, infarcts, glioses, and cortical dysplasia.

The observation that aggression associated with temporal lobe epilepsy improved postoperatively, led to the use of psychosurgery for persistently violent patients. This has provoked intense debate in Europe, Japan and the United States.

Postoperative course

Transient confusion, headache and nausea are commonly encountered immediately after operation. Incontinence of urine, rarely of faeces, may occur but only for a few days. The patient leaves the neurosurgical ward after the fifth day or so. With modern procedures, anergy, disinhibition, euphoria and excessive weight gain, all well recognised after older operations, are rarely seen.

An intensive, postoperative rehabilitation programme includes graded task assignment, aimed at the patient's resumption of family and social life, and work. Behavioural methods, like response-prevention in the obsessive/compulsive (unsuccessful before operation), can now be mounted with much better chance of success. Suicidal attempts decrease markedly following surgery; out of 66 patients admitted for stereotactic limbic leucotomy, only two subsequently killed themselves—there was doubt about a third—in the 16 months following the operation. (The expected rate of suicide in this group, without operation, is 15 per cent.)

Psychotherapy, admittedly more supportive than interpretive, may fall on less deaf ears after surgery. Whether anticonvulsants are used routinely for some months after surgery, or only with the appearance of fits, varies in different units. Epilepsy used to be seen in about 10 per cent of patients following the older, more extensive procedures. It is now encountered in about 2 per cent of patients. Outspokenness, but without emotional blunting, is noted at late follow-up in between 5 and 10 per cent of patients.

Psychotropic drugs may need to be re-introduced, if the usual indications are present. The rehabilitation period, intensive over the first 6 weeks, is carried out by enthusiastic, skilled staff who understand the needs of the patient, and are able to help him and his relatives bridge the gap between operation and homecoming. Some who find psychosurgery repellent have commented wryly that the operation is simply a licence to get well, utilising the intensive rehabilitation programme that follows. There can be no incontrovertible answer to that, though perhaps fully informed consent from the patient means an awareness of that argument too.

Conclusions

Few, faced with pressing practical problems which demand urgent answers, have the luxury of scientific certainty to help them. They do the best they can on the available evidence. The clinician has to help his patient decide on psychosurgery in as informed a way as possible.

It is clear that in intractable anxiety, depression and obsessive/compulsive disorders—and more rarely in pain—when all else has been tried and failed, relief can be obtained for a sizeable majority with present day stereotactic psychosurgical procedures.

Psychosurgery will be rendered obsolete overnight with the development of effective psychotropic medication, free of harmful effects. Perhaps the current research on synthetic endorphins will throw up such a product. In the meantime, is it beyond the bounds of possibility that some overanxious, depressed or obsessional patient may sue his doctors because the benefits of psychosurgery were not offered him earlier? The liberal conscience shudders. The demand for scientific evidence would then become insistent. Perhaps the next decade will show whether the conscience will allow the science.

FURTHER READING

Bartlett, J.R., Bridges, P.K. 1977. The extended subcaudate tractotomy lesion. In *Neuro surgical Treatment in Psychiatry, Pain and Epilepsy*. Ed. Sweet, W.H., Obrador, S. Martin Rodriguez, J.G. University Park Press. Baltimore.

Bridges, P.K., Bartlett, J.R. 1977. Review article: psychosurgery, yesterday and today. *Brit. J. Psychiatry*, **131**. 249.

Bridges, P.K. 1978. A contemporary view of psychosurgery. In *Current Themes in Psychiatry*. Ed. Gaind, R.N., Hudson, B.L. MacMillan. London.

Göktepe, E.D., Young, L.G., Bridges, P.K. 1975. A further review of the results of stereo tactic caudate trachtotomy. *Brit. J. Psychiat*. **126**. 270.

Kelly, D. 1976. Psychosurgery in the 1970s. *Brit. J. Hosp. Med.* **165**.

Metchell-Heggs, N., Kelly, D., Richardson, A. 1976. Stereotactic limbic leucotomy—a follow-up at 16 months. *Brit. J. Psychiat*. **128**. 226.

U.S. National Commission for the Protection of Human Subjects of Biomedical and Behavioural Research. 1977. *Report and Recommendations: Psychosurgery*. US DHEW Publication No. (OS) 77-001.

Robin, A., MacDonald, D. 1975. *Lessons of Leucotomy*. Henry Kimpton. London.

Valenstein, E.S. 1973. *Brain Control: A Critical Examination of Brain Stimulation and Psychosurgery*. Wiley. New York.

4

Psychotherapy and the use of drugs: narcoanalysis and abreaction

Psychotherapy is a loose term, ranging in meaning from simple supportive talk and encouragement to interpretation of a patient's behaviour and feelings, based on the concept of the dynamic unconscious. Every psychiatrist, whatever his theoretical outlook, talks to his patient, counsels him, helps him solve his problems. A patient has his depression lifted by e.c.t., but he must still resolve his marital conflicts. The university student whose schizophrenic illness has been brought under control by a phenothiazine requires help and advice to readjust, to cope with the stresses which precipitated his illness. The agoraphobic housewife whose symptoms are lifted by the use of a MAOI and behaviour therapy, needs to discuss the problems arising from her new found freedom.

Whatever treatment a patient receives, an emotional relationship inevitably springs up between him and his doctor. His attitude to his therapist influences his response to treatment. The more he likes him the more likely he is to benefit from his treatment. Psychotherapy, in this sense, accompanies all treatments.

Sometimes the therapist may wish to speed up his patient's progress, bring repressed conflicts quickly to the surface, and create an emotional situation where the patient is able to express his feelings more readily, without inhibition. To this end, he uses drugs, in narcoanalysis and excitatory abreactive techniques.

It is commonplace that under the influence of alcohol a man reveals tendencies that remain hidden in everyday life; he may become suggestible, obstinate, euphoric or boastful. Tongues are loosened by drink; critical judgment is suspended and secret aspirations, damaging confessions and dramatic falsifications of previous events come pouring out. Primitive religions have made use of such mechanisms, with an added therapeutic effect. The emotional release that occurs under alcohol and other drugs may be followed by relaxation and relief of depression. The unsophisticated man feels he has been through an experience of religious significance, that he is spiritually renewed and trouble free. Sailors, after long voyages, often feel the need of a prolonged alcoholic spree to relieve accumulated emotional tension. Psychiatry, in its turn, has discovered the value of these methods both for treatment and for exploration.

Instead of giving alcohol by mouth, the effects of which take some time to appear, and are unreliable and difficult to control, we can now employ a whole range of agents more certain in their action. Although present day drugs have reduced the demand for these they still remain useful therapeutic and diagnostic weapons; they include intravenous barbiturates and methylamphetamine, and inhalants such as ether, nitrous oxide and high percentages of carbon dioxide in oxygen.

The chief use of barbiturate abreaction is in dealing with hysterical conversion symptoms. After the precipitating event, a car crash perhaps, or the exposure of some misdeed, the individual blanches, starts to sweat and tremble, and becomes panicky. This is succeeded by hysterical conversion; amnesia, or loss of function of a limb. 'Paralysed with fright' is a far from inaccurate description. The motivated manipulation of the symptom is a mechanism which only appears some time later, when the condition has been allowed to persist. If the patient is seen at an early stage, soon after the first abrupt appearance of the symptom, intravenous injection of a barbiturate can reverse the picture. The drawn face of the patient relaxes, colour appears, and memory or full use of the limbs return without any suggestion having been made to that effect. In cases which have lasted longer, and in which the behaviour pattern has become more fixed, forceful suggestion may be required as well as the relaxing effect of the drug.

Although a patient becomes more open to suggestion and reassurance under intravenous amylobarbitone, no true hypnotic state is produced, and posthypnotic suggestion is not possible. But in both hypnosis and barbiturate narcosis there is reduction of the critical sense, an enhancement of rapport, and often a pouring out of both truth and fantasy. Aggressive feelings, which would terrify the patient in his normal state, can be expressed without excessive anxiety, and past emotional experiences lived anew.

There are no contra-indications to barbiturate narcosis, apart from those associated with barbiturates in general. Other medication does not have to be stopped.

Intravenous methylamphetamine has a different effect. Tension is heightened and the flow of talk greatly increased; the patient may bring out conflicts which have been repressed for years. Methylamphetamine can succeed in this way when the relaxing effect of barbiturates has failed. Inhibited people of obsessional disposition respond particularly well. We have used methylamphetamine with considerable effect (when other methods have failed) in psychosexual problems. The increased rapport which develops under the drug should be made use of from the beginning, and the first two or three interviews are often the vital ones.

The action of the drug is prolonged, and sometimes the patient can hardly be prevented from talking to all and sundry for some hours after the injection. Methylamphetamine is also a useful diagnostic tool, when there is doubt as to whether a patient has schizophrenia.

Other drugs, nitrous oxide, ether, and carbon dioxide are rarely used today. Nitrous oxide causes a rapid and short anaesthesia, on emerging from which abreaction in a fairly clear state of consciousness can be produced. Ether is useful in cases where some degree of excitation is required to aid abreaction. Carbon dioxide quickly brings about dissociation, and may reveal problems whose existence may not have been suspected. The psychological effects of all these drugs have much in common, and there are patients for whom each is more suitable than the others; the skill of the therapist in using them is the critical factor.

Technique with barbiturates

With hysterical conversion symptoms treatment should start as soon as possible after their appearance; the probability of success diminishes with time. The treatment should be regarded as a method of first-aid, to abolish a hysterical symptom before entrenchment and before its possible advantages are sensed by the patient. Every attempt should be made to get rid of the hysterical symptom at the first interview, and powerful suggestion may be necessary as the patient lies on the couch prepared for injection. The drug used may be sodium amylobarbitone, thiopentone or methohexitone. Choice will depend on the predilections of the clinician, but as each drug has slightly different properties, it is best to get used to one. If sodium amylobarbitone is used, 500 mg are dissolved in 10 ml distilled water. The injection is made slowly, 100 mg a minute or less being given. Conversation is continued throughout, not least in order to know the exact stage of anaesthesia reached. What is desired is a state of complete relaxation and well being, without slurring of speech or mental confusion. The dose required differs from patient to patient, and in the same patient at different times. More will be needed when he is very anxious than when calm. As emotion is aroused during the conversation further small quantities of the drug may be given to damp down anxiety, and consequent resistance to further disclosures. The full effect of each ml injected may not be apparent for a minute or two after it is given, and it is easy for the unwary to overshoot the desirable end point.

The first outward sign that the drug is starting to take effect is a heavy sigh and a change to a steadier and deeper respiration. Facial expression becomes more relaxed and friendly, and mobility returns; tears may appear. At this stage questioning becomes more direct. The doctor should gain complete control of the proceedings and quietly dominate the patient. The patient with amnesia should be questioned about his life around that time, and be brought gradually nearer the episode. Once isolated incidents have been recalled they can be used as bases for the exploration of other gaps. All the time the idea is conveyed to him that he can think more clearly, and that his memory is returning. Sometimes, especially when amnesia is of very recent onset, none of this is necessary, and memory returns of its own accord in the early stages of the injection. Sometimes blockage occurs after a large part has been regained, and this usually means that a critical traumatic incident has been reached. Then the patient is likely to display great emotion, and may need the anaesthesia to be deepened, and pressure from the doctor, before memory returns with a dramatic emotional abreaction. When the story is complete, it should be run over again and again until it can all be talked about, even if the conversation is almost sinister in its recital of harrowing experiences shorn of their appropriate affect.

The patient is unlikely to reveal vital secrets unless he is prepared to do so. It is hopeless, for instance, to expect a confession from the malingerer, who usually only becomes abusive and truculent under this treatment. A friendly emotional *rapport* must be retained throughout; 'beating up' the patient will defeat its own ends.

When memory has been restored it must be reinforced. The patient must not be allowed to go to sleep. It is wise to let the inpatient return to the ward. An hour later he may be seen again and the discussion renewed, or, as with our outpatients, a nurse takes over the conversation. Memories are then retained clearly. If the patient is allowed to go to sleep at the end of the interview, he may well forget the whole episode and the treatment will have been in vain.

Sometimes the doctor is told fantastic stories under the drug, straight from the world of nightmare. The falsity of these is often apparent, but sometimes the therapist remains unsure how much is fact or fantasy. From the point of view of therapeutic success this is unimportant, and the exploration of a patient's fantasy may release as much emotion as a real trauma, with equal effectiveness.

The same procedure is adopted when dealing with the loss of function of a limb or voice. As the drug takes effect attention is gradually directed to the affected limb. It is at first passively moved by the doctor, then the patient's more active co-operation is invited. At the end of the treatment it is important to make him exercise the limb in front of others. Once the patient finds himself committed, relapse is unlikely to occur unless he is subjected to further stress. If treatment is unsuccessful it is wise to give the patient enough drug at the end to put him to sleep, so that the interview may be forgotten or blurred when he awakes. The doctor then has to decide whether to repeat the attempt later or use another method.

Excitatory abreaction

A fundamentally different management of the abreactive technique has led to interesting and valuable results. This consists of adding to and stimulating the patient's excitement, rather than damping it down, when it often reaches a climactic phase and the patient passes into a state of temporary general inhibition. Relief from tension and hysterical symptoms, when these occur, is often very dramatic.

An excitatory abreaction can be obtained under hypnosis, and it may occur during the course of an analysis as traumatic events are uncovered. Where circumstances are favourable, it may be deliberately induced with the aid of ether, nitrous oxide or methylamphetamine.

The object of the treatment is to produce mounting excitement. Ether is probably the best drug for the purpose. It is poured on a mask and held, initially, slightly away from the patient's face. He is encouraged to start talking about past experiences which, from his history, may be expected to arouse powerful emotions, particularly those of anger and fear. As he becomes absorbed in his story the mask is brought nearer to his face. When he starts to abreact, excitement is deliberately stimulated by the therapist until the patient is shouting and struggling. At this stage nurses may be needed to hold him down; physical restraint adds to his excitement. This rises rapidly to a climax, then abruptly subsides. The patient goes limp and lies quietly for a minute or two, during which time he is unresponsive. With many patients this final stage of collapse is needed for success in treatment, and abreactions which do not go so far are ineffective. When the patient comes round his manner is composed and rational, and there is no sign of persisting excitement or intoxication. If the treatment has been successful he will then say that he feels as if a burden has been lifted from his mind.

Observations of a very similar kind were made by Pavlov on dogs. He found that they showed a similar disruption of recently formed conditioned behaviour patterns when they were excited emotionally to the point of temporary cortical inhibition. Those animals who showed signs of a constitutional instability were only made more unstable by such an experience; but in others of more stable constitution, who were subjected to the experiment, the abolition of recent conditioned patterns of behaviour permitted the return of pre-existing habits and the easier formation of new ones.

So it is with human beings. The patient who has undergone an excitatory abreaction has no doubt that something vital has occurred. The terms in which he compares his previous state of mind to his present one often bear a striking resemblance to descriptions of miraculous conversions at revivalist meetings. After the emotional storm, not only is the slate wiped clean, as it were, but the patient is left in a more impressionable state than before. Such a situation is familiar to the analyst, who can expect heightening of transference feelings when repressed emotions are abreacted by his patient. The enhanced suggestibility of the patient after abreaction can be used by the therapist to implant new ideas, and more adaptable ways of behaving. The extent to which new behaviour patterns are retained depends largely on the constitutional stability of the patient, and on the after-treatment.

This method of treatment is limited in its application. The chronically anxious patient is not helped; indeed his instability may be increased. Obsessional symptoms are rarely relieved; they are often, in fact, made worse by excitatory abreaction. Endogenously depressed patients do not respond well, and usually cannot be made to abreact. Depersonalisation may respond to abreaction only if hysterical features are apparent. It is, above all, the hysterical patient of fairly stable personality, who has broken down under severe stress, who does well with this method.

Abreactive therapy is not often needed today. In recent years we have found that patients of the kind we used to abreact respond well to other treatments, particularly MAOI and tricyclic antidepressants.

Technique with intravenous methylamphetamine

We have described the use of drugs to abolish recently implanted conversion symptoms, and to disrupt hysterical behaviour patterns by excitation. Drugs may also be used as aids in one or other of the established psychotherapeutic procedures, in which problems in the past and present life of the patient are quietly worked over. For this purpose intravenous methylamphetamine is highly effective, in spite of the bad reputation it has earned as an addictive drug through its abuse. It is of course now restricted in the UK under the Dangerous Drugs Act (1965).

Methylamphetamine is particularly useful in the treatment of certain psychosexual problems. Many patients with frightening sado-masochistic and other fantasies which are unacceptable to them are incapable, unaided, of breaking through their inhibitions and discussing freely their thoughts and feelings. Such patients are usually tense, inhibited people, with strongly obsessional personalities, too insecure to relax their rigid self-control. Under the influence of methylamphetamine their inhibitions loosen, and it becomes increasingly easy for them to discuss their difficulties and fears.

Methylamphetamine can also sometimes relieve depersonalisation, when this is secondary to an obsessional tension state. Obsessional women with long-standing anorexia nervosa are sometimes able to break out of their narrow world, bounded by food and fear of fatness, and discuss their deeper problems; but although they may relax and feel transformed for some hours, this state does not endure. Nonetheless, the experience may serve to increase their motivation and develop a positive transference, which the therapist can then utilise.

Methylamphetamine is useful diagnostically. Patients with a predominantly obsessional personality become alert, and their pulse slows under the drug's influence. In contrast, the hysterical personality is likely to feel drowsy and even fall asleep and to develop tachycardia. Schizophrenic symptoms may be brought out by the drug; a fact which is sometimes made use of when diagnosis is in doubt.

The therapist must be prepared to give the patient a full hour or more of his time. The initial dose of the drug, injected into a vein, is 15 mg, given slowly over about 3 minutes. In some patients more than 15 mg causes an almost intolerable tension, which may be difficult to control for some hours afterwards. If too small a dose is given at the first interview inhibitions are not sufficiently loosened for success, and the hope of doing so on a second occasion is the less.

The effects of methylamphetamine last many hours. After he has finished with his therapist a patient may go on talking about his most private problems with anyone present. Special precautions to safeguard him may therefore be needed. The effect of the drug may not have entirely worn off by bedtime, and a strong sedative should be prescribed to avoid a disturbed night. If a short-acting barbiturate is given, it must be remembered that there is synergistic action, so that when the sedative is taken there may be further release of repressed emotions.

It is most important not to give intravenous methylamphetamine to any patient who is taking a monoamine oxidase inhibitor, or who has been on such a drug during the preceding 3 weeks. The combination of these two drugs is dangerous, and may cause a hypertensive encephalopathy, with possibly fatal results. Nor should this treatment be readily given after the age of 50, in the presence of heart disease or hypertension, and when there is a history of cerebral aneurysm.

Carbon dioxide inhalation therapy

We have included this section more for its historical interest than as a practical treatment today. This treatment, the inhalation of 30 per cent CO_2 and 70 per cent oxygen, was used by Meduna in 1950; and as he was responsible for the earlier introduction of convulsive therapy, it understandably aroused widespread interest.

Among the patients best suited for this treatment are traumatic states with prominent hysterical dissociation. The inhalation of CO_2 by such patients often causes a vivid re-living of the traumatic episode, and loss of symptoms. In subsequent treatments this is repeated again and again until the emotions connected with the incident are finally dispersed.

Many patients are unsuitable for CO_2 treatment. Obsessional conditions are often made worse by the treatment, and anxiety states with obsessional features are also likely to be aggravated.

The treatment is safe. The amount of oxygen in the mixture ensures that the patient remains a good colour, even if 50 or more breaths are taken; cyanosis calls for an immediate stop. As with all the abreactive treatments, caution must be exercised in those over 45 years of age.

The mixture of 30 per cent CO_2 with 70 per cent oxygen is delivered from a special cylinder into a tight-fitting face-mask, with re-breathing bag and an expiratory valve to prevent a rise of pressure. The patient should not have had food for 3 hours before treatment. He lies on a couch, and is warned that as he breathes and begins to lose consciousness he will feel short of breath. Anxiety at this stage may be combated by an induction with nitrous oxide, with the switch to CO_2 when consciousness becomes clouded. If much anxiety is felt the method must be abandoned.

Psychotherapy with and without drugs

In this chapter we have described the ways in which certain drugs may be used to aid psychotherapy. The pharmacological actions of these drugs are only one part of the therapeutic picture. Often the main part they play is to induce in the patient a state of mind in which he is particularly open to psychotherapeutic procedures, whether of suggestion, exploration, or abreaction. What often matters most is the psychological impact made by the therapist on his patient during this period of susceptibility. It is clear that psychoanalysis scores its greatest successes in those very patients who are also most readily helped by drug aided pyschotherapy, such as we have described above. The same qualitative changes can be observed with both methods of treatment; increase of transference, abreaction, the breaking up of old patterns of thought and the implantation of new ones, even an increase in 'insight'. To be sure, the degree of 'insight' registered will depend on the theoretical opinions of the therapist, and the extent to which he is convinced that the patient has adopted his own view of the case.

Drug aided psychotherapy is not successful with graver states any more than psychoanalysis is; schizophrenia and endogenous depressions, severe anxiety states and obsessional neuroses, for which more specific methods are required.

FURTHER READING

Sargant, W. 1957. *Battle for the mind.* Heinemann, London.

5

Behavioural psychotherapy

Most people at some time in their lives are able to change themselves; how they behave, their habits, how they think and feel. Some stop smoking; some learn to control their over-reaction to anxiety or anger; some improve their social graces. But sometimes undesirable behaviour persists in spite of every attempt by the individual to help himself; and eventually outside help may be sought.

Behavioural psychotherapy utilises modern theories of learning to help people rid themselves of undesirable behaviour, and to replace this with one that is more satisfactory, not only to the individual but often to others. The term 'behaviourist' has unfortunate connotations. Behavioural psychotherapy does not simply concern itself with behaviour. It also embraces cognitions, emotions and, perhaps less successfully, volition. Its concern is not only with people's activities but also with their experience; with the washing rituals of an obsessive/compulsive patient, the terror of the phobic individual, the depressive's gloomy evaluation of his existence and future, and his tendency to shun all satisfying activities.

Behavioural psychotherapy revolves around two apparently simple notions:

1. When two events occur together in time, they become linked in the mind. This is, of course, the basic principle of classical conditioning. The hungry dog salivates when offered food. If a buzzer goes off at the same time, sooner or later the dog salivates when he hears the buzzer alone.

2. Those activities which are pleasurable are more likely to be repeated than those which are not (operant conditioning).

Behavioural psychotherapy conjures up the spectre of a powerful technology capable of almost anything; in totalitarian institutions, of brainwashing. In reality, the successes of behavioural psychotherapy are modest. The initial reports of near 100 per cent success have given way to more realistic estimates of its therapeutic value.

Behavioural and interpretive psychotherapists have been equally contemptuous of each other's efforts in the past. Behaviourists have mocked the search for meaning of those who look for insight in psychotherapy. The believe that non-specific elements in the relationship between patient and therapist are more important than the belief system of interpretive psychotherapists. The latter, in their turn, see behavioural psychotherapists' pre-occupation with conscious experience and observable activity as blinkered. The combativeness of the two therapeutic approaches is passing and a rapprochment is under way. Therapists of both schools are seeking to understand, within their own conceptual frameworks, what the others are doing. They are trying to enhance the effectiveness of treatment by borrowing from each other's methods. The agoraphobic may find insights in interpretive psychotherapy which she cannot use, to make travel to and from her behavioural therapist possible. An action-orientated intervention, with exposure in vivo for example, may free her to use the public transport system and allow her to continue her quest for meaning with her interpretive psychotherapist. The injection-phobic may allow her behavioural psychotherapist to hover for hours over the antecubital vein with needle and syringe, when an interpretive intervention could suddenly facilitate the dreaded puncture.

It might be asked why behaviour therapies feature in a book on physical methods of treatment in psychiatry. There are several reasons. The methods of treatment are often so physical themselves; the self-shocking of the paedophile, as he attempts to control his fantasies or illegal activities, has an obvious physical component. Persuading an agoraphobic to enter a lift or tube-train, to help her habituate to the confined situation, may at times necessitate physical containment, as well as psychological understanding. The entire field of biofeedback depends on converting unconscious physiological events into signals. Another reason relates to the interaction between drugs and behaviour therapies. Psychopharmacology has much the same objectives as behavioural psychotherapy. It aims at modulating emotions, changing cognitions, and altering what the patient actually does. It is not surprising that psychopharmacological and behavioural psychotherapeutic means have been combined. The use of short-acting barbiturates intravenously to facilitate desensitisation to phobic stimulation, of anxiolytics and beta blockers in exposure therapy, of monoamine oxidase inhibitors in diminishing phobic avoidance and panic, and of clomipramine combined with behavioural methods in the treatment of the obsessive-compulsive, are examples.

What then happens between the patient and the behavioural psychotherapist?

BEHAVIOURAL ANALYSIS

The patient, unable to help himself despite encouragement and aid from friends and relations, comes for therapy, often with a sense of shame. The behaviour therapist's first task is to delineate in detail the size and shape of the problem presented. This has been called the behavioural analysis; with feelings and cognitions subsumed under that heading. The *sequence* of actions, emotions, and thoughts complained of by the patient, is elicited in detail, together with the changes wanted. A search is made for what precedes the sequence and what follows it, what originated it in the past, and what seems to be maintaining it in the present.

A business man had been drinking heavily in the evenings for over 7 years. He was in his early fifties, and further promotion in his organisation was unlikely. Younger and abler men were surpassing him. His son had dropped out of university, and openly criticised him. His wife was irritated and bored by him, and their sexual relationship had ended years ago, partly because of his drinking.

His drinking was confined to the early evening, but was rapid and continued to drunkenness. Reasonable conversation was only possible with his wife and son in the early stages. Verbal violence developed later, usually during the evening meal. This was succeeded by heavy sleep, often on the floor. The patient awoke in the early hours, remorseful, with no desire for alcohol. He went to bed, but remained wakeful and fretful until dawn, when sleep supervened; just before he had to face another day, an alienated family, and a competitive work situation with which he could now barely cope.

Any behavioural approach that disregarded the complex problems apparent above is not likely to succeed for long.

THERAPY OBJECTIVES

An important feature of behavioural psychotherapy is the defining of a specific aim of treatment agreed on by patient and therapist; the therapeutic target. This has the advantage of forcing patient and therapist, and outsiders, to assess progress and ultimately to see whether the target has been achieved or not. A patient with a dog phobia may set herself the objective of stroking a neighbour's terrier for 5 minutes. An obsessional may aim to reduce hand washing from 80 to less than 7 times a day, with no wash to last more than a minute. An exhibitionist may aim to masturbate in his room without his 'hunt-flash-masturbate-escape' sequence.

Baseline levels of the activities, emotions and cognitions that are involved in therapy are recorded, often graphically for visual impact. For example, the number of deviant urges, fantasies and actions may be charted by the fetishist alongside his more normal sexual activity. It is against this baseline—and recording it may have its own impact on behaviour—that the results of treatment are charted.

MOTIVATION FOR CHANGE

The patient and therapist have understandably been evaluating each other during the behavioural analysis and objective-setting. The therapist's competence, trustworthiness, confidence in his methods, interest, perhaps even humanity, are scrutinised by the patient. The therapist, alongside his other tasks, has been trying to estimate the motivation and capacity for change of his patient and, where possible, to heighten it.

If the question, 'Why do you want to change?', is answered by 'To be more normal', the therapist has reason to be uneasy. The wish for more specific advantages to be derived from changes in the direction targetted carry greater hopes of success. Many therapists outline in unsparing detail the steps that therapy can take, and assess the patient's motivation from how he receives this.

Action change

Activity acquisition

When the problem is to help the patient behave in a *new* way, the therapist must be sure that the patient is *capable* of this. A patient may be highly anxious under certain social circumstances. His anxiety may interfere with his social behaviour and conceal the fact that this is reasonably sophisticated. By contrast, another man may be markedly deficient in this field. Deficiency in social skills may exist irrespective of social anxiety; for example, in the mentally handicapped or chronically institutionalised patient. Therapy may be either on an individual basis or in groups, but in both events encourages the patients to develop those roles they habitually fear and shirk. Some patients find it difficult to assert themselves. They behave passively, and are liable to be bullied by other people; and occasionally they explode inappropriately.

Subnormals and schizophrenics, who lack basic social skills, are helped by rehearsing increasingly sophisticated social roles with the therapist, or in groups. Other members of a social skills group may contribute to this process, perhaps modelling for the patient appropriate ways of dealing with whatever situation is presented. Modelling, as well as feedback on the patient's own performance, is an important part of therapy, as is the therapist's approval of desirable activities in the patient. The whole procedure may be enriched by the use of video tape. The patient's behaviour can be reviewed and commented on, not least by the patient himself.

Role rehearsal can be supplemented by *role reversal*. A simple example is provided by the patient who is reluctant, through timidity, to return a pair of defective shoes to the shop and ask for his money back. He first of all rehearses several ways of approaching the shopkeeper; then he himself assumes the role of the shopkeeper. This gives the patient a wider view of the problem and allows him to modify his behaviour and develop self confidence. Ultimately, play activity must be replaced by the real life task of actually returning a pair of shoes to the shop. Some social skills groups have actually bought goods in order to return them to the shop, to enable patients to acquire the self confidence that, up until now, has eluded them.

Activity increase

When a patient performs some necessary action only very infrequently—and reluctantly—an increase of this activity may become the objective of therapy. In marital therapy, for example, conducted on behavioural lines, the couple may describe activities that they wish to encourage in each other. The wife wants more talk about the events of her husband's day when he arrives home in the evening. The husband expects a greater show of affection when he comes through the door. Each partner draws up a list of changes he and she would like to see in the other. Exchanges are then agreed upon, each item in the husband's list being matched by one in his wife's. Charts are kept of the frequency of such agreed activities. These are not discussed between sessions, but are examined with the therapist who, in his objective role, can constructively point out the deficiencies of one or both the couple.

Sometimes the increase in desirable behaviour also requires changes in its nature. This may be helped by the use of what is known as *shaping*. The final target is approached by a series of ever-nearer approximations, each stage being rewarded and therefore reinforced when attained. A self-charted record of the patient's progress, combined with his therapist's approval or otherwise, may be sufficient.

Token economy, which is based on shaping, has been extensively used to increase the range and desirability of the activities of many patients; for example, in the rehabilitation of chronic schizophrenics. Treatment objectives are set for individual patients, designed to start 'from where the patient is at'. When unwanted activities are reduced and replaced by more suitable behaviour, tokens are given. They are exchanged in the ward shop for cigarettes, sweets, beverages and items of clothing.

Alongside reward and punishment, *aversion relief* therapy has a useful part to play. When an unpleasant stimulus stops, the patient feels pleasurable relief. The unpleasant stimulus can be terminated by a patient himself, under the right circumstances. For instance, a paedophile is sexually aroused by the picture of a child. He receives continuous, aversive electrical stimulation, via his forearm, during the showing of the photograph. This can be ended at any time by his substituting the slide of a reasonably attractive (for him) adult for that of the child, with immediate relief from discomfort.

Activity decrease

Habit disorders may involve any one or more of a number of undesirable activities; smoking, drinking, overeating, hair pulling, nose picking, are examples. Only by understanding the situations and factors that contribute to such behaviour can the patient and therapist construct a realistic therapeutic plan of action.

Consider, for instance, a patient with alcoholism. The amount drunk, and when, is delineated. Given reasonable motivation it is sometimes possible to reduce significantly the amount drunk by altering the patient's drinking ritual; alcohol may be drunk in an unusual room, from a less attractive glass or container, and in a less pleasant form, absinthe say, instead of gin. The approval of his spouse, his workmates, his therapist, when he stays clear of alcohol, or strictly controls his drinking, enhances the patient's morale and self-respect.

Biofeedback techniques, utilising blood levels of alcohol (from apparatus like the breathalyser), may be used in the training of chronic alcoholics who are unwilling to become completely teetotal. The knowledge that their blood alcohol has not risen above, say, 60 mg per cent during a sociable evening both encourages and trains them to keep their drinking within clearcut limits. Exceeding the agreed intake may carry a *response-cost* in the shape of some self-imposed deprivation. A donation of money to a charity is sometimes used as a penalty.

Where total abstinence is the objective, some form of conditioning may be tried. It is comparatively easy to associate an electrical stimulus in time with the smell or taste of a favourite alcoholic drink. It need not be particularly painful and can be self-administered. The objective is to couple an unpleasant sensation with the drink, and to develop an avoidance response. Ampomorphine induces nausea and vomiting, and may be similarly paired with the alcoholic drink. It requires medical personnel for the injection and its timing is less precise than electrical stimulation, but it is more effective (see p. 151). The induction of a terrifying paralysis by intravenous scoline immediately after the patient has poured himself a drink and taken a sip is another, although rarely used, method.

Self-regulatory techniques include *covert sensitisation.* The patient imagines the shameful consequences of his undesirable actions; the alcoholic sees the dead victim of his drunken driving and the consequences; the paedophile conjures up pictures of prison and his family's shame.

Activity loss

In successfully treated cases a steady decrease in unwanted activities is succeeded by their total disappearance. A paedophile, for example, heterosexual or homosexual, well motivated, may come for treatment. After baseline charting, electrical shock aversion, using paedophilic images and photographs, may start the treatment. Alternatively, sexual arousal, initially induced by slides and pictures of children, may be coupled with showing pictures of sexually attractive adults of the preferred sex. The procedure of *fading* aims gradually to increase the arousing properties of adults and to decrease that of children. Any deficiency of social skills in the paedophile relating to dating or mating behaviour must be rectified. The effect of the patient's behaviour on his family and friends must be understood, and appropriate measures, where indicated, undertaken. When behavioural psychotherapy alone is not successful in such cases, reduction in sexual interest may be achieved by use of drugs; butyrophenone, benperidol, or the antiandrogen, cyproterone (see p. 131).

Obsessive/compulsive rituals, which are often concerned with contamination and harm, have been reduced by *response-prevention*. In this form of therapy, the anxiety which is aroused when the patient is unable to complete his senseless ritual is prolonged, so that ultimately it is reduced and extinguished. The drive to perform the compulsive behaviour is thereby lessened.

Cognition change

Increasingly, behavioural psychotherapy looks for help from the patient's imagery, thoughts and beliefs. Observable behaviour is properly seen as only part of human activity and experience.

Ellis has pioneered what he calls 'rational emotive therapy'. He proposed an ABC model. C is the unwanted activity or emotional state the patient wishes to discard. Inquiry is made as to the circumstance, or event, A, which produces this feeling state or activity. B is the irrational linking belief which therapy aims to change. For example, if A is a forthcoming examination, and C is the anxiety associated with it, the belief, B, may include a considerable underestimation by the patient of his preparedness for the examination, and of his intellectual abilities. He may have unrealistic ideas of the attitudes of the examiners, and of the standards expected of candidates. The aim of therapy is to counter such distorted beliefs; in effect, to change the language he uses as he faces the problem.

Meichenbaum has extensively explored inner language, attempting to get patients to think positively, to substitute a coping language in their own words for the non-coping, defeatist language they use to describe various fear-inducing situations. The latter are delineated, as usual, in the behavioural analysis. The patient then learns to express his thoughts, both to himself and others, in more realistic terms. He makes less awesome predictions about the outcome, focusses on his strengths rather than assumed weaknesses, and reminds himself of past successes. He substitutes a 'but language' (I feel panicky *but* I will cope) for an 'and language' (I feel panicky *and* I will pass out).

Emotion change

The management of emotions by changing inner language has also been applied to the self control of anger and depression. A coping, managing language is fashioned, away from the anger producing circumstances, but for use later within them. Repeated, carping criticism, from a colleague at work, for instance, can be coolly disregarded with the prepared, but obviously credible thought that, 'his fault-finding is necessary to bolster his low self confidence; he's an inadequate man.'

The repetitive self-denigrations of the depressive need to be supplanted by increasingly confident and positive thinking. This can be encouraged by linking positive thinking to common everyday activities, such as drinking, smoking or eating. (The Premack principle states that low frequency activities multiply when repeatedly coupled with high frequency ones.) The patient must repeat to himself that he is capable, likeable, has good prospects for the future, and so on, whenever he starts and finishes a cigarette, a drink or a meal.

The treatment of phobic anxiety invariably requires some form of exposure to the phobic stimulus. This may be imagined, or occur in real life circumstances. Either exposure may be made in a graded fashion, moving from the least to the most terrifying aspects of the situation or object which is feared, or it may happen rapidly by immediate confrontation with the most terrifying elements in the hierarchy.

Imaginal desensitisation, with or without a relaxation procedure, involves imagining items in a hierarchy, starting with the least terrifying; when an item can be thought of without anxiety, the patient moves to the next one. This 'within-the-head' exposure therapy allows the patient to habituate to the induced anxiety, and thus learn to adapt better. He is able to develop his own, more realistic language, without the tuition required by the Meichenbaum approach.

The *graded exposure in vivo* of the phobic patient starts with real life encounters which he can barely tolerate. He gradually habituates to the anxiety, and proves to himself that his fearful predictions are only shadows. As fear steadily decreases he climbs the hierarchical tree, until eventually he can face the situation which previously most terrified him. The agoraphobic who has managed to walk from his home to the bus stop, with consequently decreasing anxiety, may now find it comparatively easy to catch a bus and stay on it, terminus to terminus, until he no longer feels in the least anxious. Travel by underground train may now become possible.

Intravenous methohexitone sodium, a rapidly acting, short-lived barbiturate may help a patient face dreaded situations. As its effect wears off, and the patient stays in the phobic situation, the opportunity occurs to habituate on exposure. Diazepam, but only if blood levels of the drug are waning, also enhances the effect of exposure. The last dose should be taken no closer than 3 hours before the exposure exercise.

The imaginary confrontation of the most terrifying items in the phobic patient's hierarchy is called *implosion*. Sometimes the therapist provides a fear-inducing narrative, but in general it is better to let the patient provide one for himself, for this is bound to be more realistic and terrifying to him. He describes his story in the present tense, and the therapist prompts and keeps him to the task, and does not allow him to deviate from his fearful path. The narrative is prolonged until the patient becomes habituated to his anxiety. This exposure has then of course to be tested, as does any imaginal method, in real circumstances.

Flooding in vivo is the real life confrontation by a patient of what he most fears. It is only for the most determined of patients.

It is often better to start treatment of a seriously phobic patient with phenelzine and a tranquilliser, provided the patient's personality is a reasonable one and there are no psychopathic features, or other contraindications. These drugs have the effect of gradually reducing anxiety, improving the patient's morale and self confidence, and allowing him perhaps to assert himself more at home, even venturing a few steps further afield than usual.

At the same time, a psychotherapeutic approach aims to encourage the patient to examine the deeper nature of his fears, to explore his relationship with his spouse and family, and discuss his desire and potential for development. The spouse, or parent may also be seen, alone or with the patient, and their capacity for change and adaptation assessed and utilised. At this point, some form of exposure therapy may be valuable.

The MAOI and tranquillisers controlling anxiety and accompanying autonomic symptoms need to be continued during the period of desensitisation, and for a variable time subsequently. When an agoraphobic patient has been virtually housebound for many years, he has numerous habits to break before he can be considered to be fully recovered, and able to lead a full life. In some cases, when say, neither patient nor spouse are prepared to adapt realistically to changed circumstances, drug therapy may need to be continued for years, perhaps indefinitely. Many others need a tranquilliser from time to time to cope with periodic upsurges of anxiety, which may cause maladaptive patterns to reappear.

BIOFEEDBACK TECHNIQUES

Biofeedback is the conversion of changes in physiological functions into perceptible signals. This information is then used by motivated patients to alter the physiological function in the direction desired.

A great deal of interest and apparatus has surrounded attempts to control heart rate and rhythm, blood pressure, electromyographic and electroencephalographic activity, and skin temperature. Inflated claims have been made for the control of cardiac arrhythmias and epileptic fits, the alleviation of migraine, tension headaches, anxiety and insomnia. The induction of a so-called 'alpha state', comparable to that found in meditation, by training alpha rhythms on the e.e.g., has been claimed. Controlled trails have been few, though it must be said that sham feedback has, on the whole, been less helpful than true feedback in the conditions mentioned. Blood pressure has been reduced 'to a statistically but not clinically significant' level (by about 10 mm Hg) in hypertensives. No doubt the present day intense research activity will eventually show just what place the modality has in therapy. At the time of writing, its contribution seems unlikely to be large.

CRITICISMS OF BEHAVIOURAL PSYCHOTHERAPY

Three main themes can be seen in the criticisms levelled against behavioural psychotherapy. The first is that it is too powerful and inhuman a technology; its future development must be watched with care. The second is that it is too weak to be relevant to human difficulties, because it deals only with symptoms and not with causes; symptom-elimination will simply be followed by symptom-substitution. The third is that the results of behavioural psychotherapy are further proof of the gullibility and suggestibility of some human beings at the hands of others.

The power of behavioural psychotherapy has been overestimated, not least by therapists themselves. Initial 'cure' rates above the 90 per cent mark have, in recent years, been replaced by more moderate claims of success in individuals who are 'sufficiently motivated' for change. The counter-controls a person can exert over his would-be therapist are great in any free situation. Even in the total-control situation of prison and prisoner-of-war camps, few adult brains were, and are, lastingly brainwashed.

Behavioural psychotherapists do not find it necessary to conceptualise the actions and experiences they try to change as 'symptoms' of some underlying conflict or illness. Change is rarely followed by new unwanted substitute behaviour. No new decontaminating or other ritual replaces hand-washing in the obsessional. Relapse, on the other hand, is not uncommon, and booster sessions to maintain earlier treatment gains are often needed.

Although symptom substitution is not a serious problem, it needs to be said that the cure of a patient may create difficulties in those closely involved with him or her. For instance, hostility and jealousy may develop or increase in the husbands of agoraphobic wives, as the latter improve. They become insecure and alarmed as their wives become more independent. The therapist who is aware of this possibility will take steps to deal with this at an early stage of treatment.

The third criticism suggests that the nonspecific aspects of the transactions between patient and therapist are more important than the therapeutic. The hope of the patient, self confidence of the therapist, his interest in his patient, the nature of the relationship they build, are, on this view, the essential elements of therapy. Most so-called controlled studies in behavioural psychotherapy fail to allow for the therapist's and patient's belief in the efficacy of the treatment. If, together, they achieve results they both appreciate, that would seem to be justification enough. If such a result can be further enhanced by the use of medication or interpretive psychotherapy, who would sacrifice therapeutic gain for ideology?

FURTHER READING

Bandura, A. 1969. *Principles of Behaviour Modification*. Holt, Rheinhart & Winston. New York.

Beech, H.R. 1978. Advances in the treatment of obsessional neurosis. *Brit. J. Hosp. Med.* **19**. 54.

Falloon, I.R.H., Lindley, P., MacDonald R., Marks, I.M. 1977. Social skills training of outpatients. A controlled study of rehearsal and homework. *Brit. J. Psychiat.* **31**. 599.

Meichenbaum, D. 1974. *Cognitive Behaviour Modification*. N. J. General Learning Press. Morristown.

Rachman, S. 1976. The modification of obsessions: A new formulation. *Behav. Research Therapy*. **14**. 437.

Seligman, M.E.P. 1974. Depression and learned helplessness. In *Handbook of Behaviour Modification and Behaviour Therapy*. Ed. H. Leitenberg. Englewood Cliff. New Jersey.

6

Psychosomatic medicine

The study of psychosomatic disease—or psychophysiologic disorders—is little more than half a century old. Disorders such as asthma, neurodermatitis, peptic ulcer, ulcerative colitis, hypertension, coronary artery disease, and rheumatoid arthritis were at one time said to be typical examples of psychosomatic disease, in which emotions played a decisive role, acting through the autonomic nervous system. Much of the early work was inspired by psychoanalytic thought. Deutsch put forward the idea of 'organ neurosis', part of the body sensitised from early years to react to emotional conflicts. Dunbar suggested that there were specific personality types associated with different psychosomatic diseases. Alexander postulated that specific psychodynamic conflicts resulted in certain definite diseases. The peptic ulcer patient, for example, was seen as having a 'dependency conflict', a powerful but ambivalent desire for love, equated with food, the conflict arising from early dissatisfactions at the breast. An anxiety-provoking situation later in life re-evoked the specific conflict over dependency and (in high pepsinogen secretors) an ulcer was formed; but while many peptic ulcer patients do show such passive dependent conflicts, many others do not. Theories of specificity failed to find confirmation from later research work, and perhaps even more important, no therapeutic benefit accrued for patients. Interest moved away from psychoanalytic ideas to epidemiology, behavioural psychology, psychosocial studies and psychophysiology. No longer is the view held that psychosomatic disorders have a specific single cause. Current beliefs are that a multiplicity of causes are present in most diseases, and that the various factors summate at the final common pathway.

Lipowski defines psychosomatic medicine as, in part, the science of the interaction of psychological, physiological and social factors in disease, in part an attitude to the whole person, together with those activities he calls consultation-liaison psychiatry. His model is one of information-processing by the individual. Happenings become information, which are then filtered and screened in the central nervous system, appraised and, if need be, given meaning and feeling, with appropriate autonomic and endocrine concomitants. If of high intensity, this may justify the description 'stressor' to describe the environmental event or situation. Visceral sensations, such as palpitations, are added to the information input. So too is the subject's appraisal of his capacity to cope, and of the social support available to him to diminish the effect of the stress. If these are inadequate, the hypothesis runs, the individual becomes susceptible to disease.

Exactly what disease develops depends on (1) the presence of a pathogen, and/or (2) an organ, or organ system vulnerability, innate or acquired. Organ vulnerability may be some analogue of autonomic specificity. It is well known that when anxious, some people develop tachycardia, others get headaches, diarrhoea, or frequency of micturition, yet others outwardly unperturbed have anxiety 'come out of their arm pits'.

The proposition that liability to illness follows inability to counter stress effectively has links with Selye's work on the general adaptation syndrome, with its successive phases of alarm, adjustment and exhaustion. The cluster syndrome of Hinckle and Wolff, that half of all illness occurs in a third of all people, and that illness of all sorts follows 'unsatisfactory years', is another facet of the same notion. It has received support from 'life events' research; much of which is, admittedly, retrospective and open to bias of patient and researcher. The common finding is of a crescendo of life events—bereavement, job loss, marital separation, illness in the family—in the period leading up to the illness under investigation: myocardial infarction, depression, schizophrenia, subarachnoid haemorrhage, accidents and so on. Prospective studies have been few and difficult to do, but have mostly shown modest, positive correlations between event-reporting and subsequent illness.

Experimental work with animals subjected to psychosocial stress has demonstrated the emergence of physical disease. Rats raised in unusually crowded circumstances not only fight more but also develop hypertension and arteriolar changes. Whether sustained essential hypertension in man can be similarly produced is to date unknown.

Sifneos has described 'alexithymia', and suggested that this personality characteristic is often present in psychosomatic patients. They have difficulty in expressing or describing their feelings, and may indeed be totally lost for words in this respect. There is little or no elaboration of fantasy in their emotional lives. It is alleged that an intolerable affect results, and that this in turn leads to physiological dysfunction. However, in practice there is likely to be found a graded dimension of personality, between those who have few words and those who have many for their emotions. Quantitation of this personality dimension is at present under way.

No matter what future research findings are in the physical, psychological and social areas, they are unlikely to alter radically the way in which practising clinicians investigate and set about treating their patients. Adverse life happenings, including illness itself, are likely to have occurred. The patient's defensive and coping strategies have been sorely challenged. Support from kin and friends may have failed, or been inadequate in the patient's eyes. The patient's state of mind is as much a feature of his illness as are the physical aspects. In the threat-dominated mental state, anxiety and apprehension are likely to be all pervasive. When a sense of loss dominates the patient's thoughts, depression, anger and hostility are more apparent, but depression and anxiety frequently co-exist, and it is rare to find 'pure' states. How a patient presents is therefore often complex and far from straightforward. Some patient's see their problems as primarily psychological, but more often than not physical symptoms dominate the clinical picture and the patient's thinking.

A common presentation is with unrecognised somatic features of anxiety and/or depression; palpitations, muscle discomfort, tremor, sweating and the hyper-ventilation syndrome. Gastro-intestinal symptoms, with loss of appetite, weight and energy, due to depression, may masquerade as neoplastic disease. At the same time it is essential for the clinician to remain on his toes and remember that neoplasia and depression can co-exist. He must always reassure himself that he has not overlooked some serious organic disease. Only when he has done this is he in a position to set about reassuring his patient and allay the hypochondriacal concern that is frequently present.

The distress of established physical illness is frequently heightened by the patient's dysphoric state. Twenty-five per cent of seriously ill patients on general wards, for instance, were found in one study to be measurably depressed; a figure which accords with our own findings. This often goes unnoticed in a busy ward, and declares itself circuitously in non-compliance with prescribed regimes, ill-advised self-discharge, or simply failure to improve as expected.

Recurring illness like asthma, neurodermatitis, or ulcerative colitis may be complicated by anxiety and depression. It is never easy to be sure which is chicken and which is egg, but in practice both physical disease and emotional upset need to be treated. The patient needs to be reassured, and his fears about the future discussed realistically but sensibly. Since this inevitably concerns close relatives, it is wise to involve them in the patient's treatment from an early stage. Psychotherapy is often ineffective until anxiety has been reduced to a reasonable level by anxiolytics, or the patient's despair has been relieved to some extent by an antidepressant.

The practice of psychosomatic medicine always involves the delineation along physical, psychological and sociological dimensions of the causes, features and management of a patient's symptoms and distress. The issue is no longer whether or not there are such dimensions for any problem, but how great the contribution of each is to the disorder, how much one or other can be modified to help the patient. The dimensions of course are for convenience of conceptualisation and study. The whole person is affected more or less simultaneously along all three. The physical treatments that are the subject of this book all have concurrent psychological and social effects.

Myocardial infarction, sometimes followed by angina of effort, can be used to exemplify the model and to show the place of physical treatment in its total management.

Physical contributions to its causation like smoking, beta-lipoproteinaemia, and hypertension are too well known to need recapitulation. Their predictive power is low, and there has been an intensive search for contributory psychosocial factors. Suspected sociological influences have included urbanisation, geographical and social mobility, and status incongruity. This last is a measure not of social class (whose association with ischaemic heart disease is obscure) but of incongruity between parameters of a person's standing in society. These were, in an American study, education, occupation, income, house, neighbourhood, religion and membership of voluntary societies. Good education with a low income, plus a deteriorating house in a well-to-do neighbourhood, would indicate high status incongruity. It is the incongruity, rather than any one parameter, that appears to correlate with ischaemic heart disease. Job dissatisfaction, with either too much or too little *perceived* responsibility at work, also appears to heighten risk.

Personality studies have particularly highlighted the ambitious, aggressive, competitive, time-pressured Type A behaviour pattern, which is associated with a high risk of coronary artery disease in contrast to Type B behaviour. Life changes requiring adjustment were found to double above base-line rates in the 6 months before myocardial infarction in Swedish and Finnish studies, and to quadruple if the myocardial infarction was a fatal one. Life events of predesignated magnitude that were societally imposed on the individual, or 'acts of God', clustered significantly in the 3 weeks before the attack in men aged 30 to 65 who survived a myocardial infarction. Bereavement in widowers over 55 carries a 40 per cent increased mortality risk from cardiovascular disease in the ensuing 6 months.

Preventive efforts may be in the physical sphere, by reducing smoking, blood pressure, beta-lipoproteins, and perhaps by jogging. Social measures include such steps as improving support after bereavement, and psychologically by modifying Type A behaviour, persuading the patient to change to a Type B way of life.

Myocardial infarction not only has well known physical features, pain, arrhythmias, hypotension, and so on, but important psychosocial ones. Possible loss of earnings and the relinquishing of social roles while the patient is ill inevitably increase the patient's difficulties in coming to terms with and adapting to his illness. The decision to hospitalise or not after myocardial infarction should be weighed on social as well as medical grounds. For many patients there is little or no survival advantage in admission to a coronary care unit.

Management of the infarction and its sequelae must be along physical, social and psychological lines. Rehabilitation from the illness depends on a number of factors. Lower paid men, especially with previously poor work records, overestimate the disability due to angina or heart failure, and return to work only after prolonged absence. It is all too easy for them to assume the 'sick role' and use this to compensate for their various inadequacies. The self-employed, by contrast, return early to work and underestimate the disability compared with their physician's judgment.

Medication to combat arrhythmias, angina and heart failure may need supplementation by anxiolytics and/or antidepressants. The closer the psychiatric state is to the 'endogenous' depressive profile the more likely it is to respond to a tricyclic or quadracyclic antidepressant, but care is required in this respect, due to the side effects of these drugs. Doxepin, dothiepin, mianserin, and nomifensine have so far achieved no evil reputation with regard to cardio-toxicity, and are first choice in the wake of a myocardial infarction, even though their antidepressant effects are low compared say to amitriptyline (see p. 18). Occasionally depression may be so severe that e.c.t is required. An agitated seriously suicidal patient cannot be left too long without e.c.t., although an interval of at least 6 weeks after the infarct is desirable, but the decision to go ahead with e.c.t. at any time must always depend on the balance of risks, between the possibility of causing a fatal arrhythmia and the dangers of the patient harming himself, either deliberately or through adverse neuroendocrine effects on the heart itself. Reactive depression, often with phobic features associated with left submammary chest pain and cardiac neurosis, is a not uncommon sequelae of infarction, and may respond well to one of the MAOI (see p. 21).

Anxiety-heightening times that need special help are the move from the coronary care unit to a general ward, and the period shortly after the hospital is left behind. Patients who are given a firm outpatient appointment are much less likely to become disturbed and anxious than those sent home without a definite one. Many patients, and their spouses, fear that coitus may be harmful, even fatal, and virtually abandon sexual activities. Advice on its resumption, and indeed its advisability, is often important and welcomed. Death in coitus is rare, and when it does occur is usually in unfamiliar surroundings, with an unfamiliar partner. However, if sexual adjustment was previously poor, one or other partner may well use the infarction as an excuse for steadfastly refusing to resume intercourse.

Return to former employment, or some modification of it, is the usual aim unless recovery is very incomplete. Most patients are able to return to work reasonably soon, and anyone unable to do so, say, within 6 months of a myocardial infarction, is more likely to be disabled for psychological rather than cardiac reasons. Adjustment to enforced retirement usually needs considerable psychological assistance, particularly for a patient for whom work has been the most important element in his life.

Pain

Pain may arise unassociated with a demonstrable organic cause, or be of far greater intensity than can be explained by the physical lesion present. Such pains include headache, facial pains, left submammary pain, abdominal pain, with or without the irritable bowel syndrome, musculoskeletal pain, especially in the back, and stump and/or phantom pain after limb amputation. More than 50 per cent of patients attending gastroenterological clinics for the investigation of abdominal pain have no structural lesion found to account for their complaints.

A detailed history from the patient, and preferably from at least one close relative or friend, allows the mental state to be evaluated, and the contributory factors, recent and remote, to be assessed. The characteristics, timing, antecedents, and consequences of the pain, not only to the patient but also to those around him, are established; a 'pain diary' may be of help during the early stages of investigation. The absence of an adequate physical cause must be confirmed, if necessary after appropriate investigations, and in consultation with colleagues. Many patients are taking large amounts of analgesics, including alcohol, when first seen. Quantities are determined, for not only may these drugs paradoxically be contributing to the patient's discomfort and dysphoria, but success in subsequent treatment can in part be measured by reduction in their consumption.

Thoroughness in this appraisal contributes to an informed treatment strategy and engages the patient in the therapeutic task ahead. Particularly when pain has been present for some time (see p. 21 for an account of atypical facial pain), an antidepressant drug may effect a 'miracle', rapidly diminishing or even removing the pain. It is unreasonable to expect a patient who has had pain in the face say, for several years, and who has already probably seen numerous practitioners without any relief, to accept that pain is psychological, an expression of depression and resentment, however apparent this may be to the psychiatrist. Once some relief has been achieved, however, (and we recognise that some degree of placebo effect is often present) the patient is ready to respond to a psychotherapeutic approach, to accept that his pain may reflect his feelings and relationships. Now family and friends may also need to be involved.

FURTHER READING

Birley, J.L.T., Connolly, J. 1979. Life events and physical illness. In *Modern Trends in Psychosomatic Medicine* – 3. Ed. Hill, O.W. Butterworth. London.

Brown, G.W., Harris, T. 1978. *Social Origins of Depression*. Tavistock Publication. London.

Jenkins, T.D. 1976. Recent evidence supporting psychological and social risk factors for coronary disease. *New Engl. J. Med.* **24**. 987–994 and 1033–1038.

Kimball, C.P. 1979. Reactions to illness: the acute phase. In *Symposium on Liaison Psy chiatry*. Ed. Kimball, C.P. Psychiatric Clinics of North America. W.B. Saunders Co. Philadelphia.

Lipowski, Z.J. 1977. Psychosomatic medicine in the 70s: an overview. *Amer. J. Psychiat.* **134**. 233–244.

Sternbach, R.A. 1977. Psychophysiology of pain. In *Psychosomatic Medicine*. Eds. Lipowski, Z.J., Kipsit, D.R. Whybrow, P.C. Oxford University Press. New York.

7

Weight problems: treatment of anorexia, anorexia nervosa, and obesity

Loss and gain of weight is a common feature of many illnesses, mental and physical. It may be an early sign of an affective disorder, when weight loss can be extreme. But sometimes bouts of compulsive eating develop and the patient, usually a middle-aged women with neurotic depression or a young women recovering from anorexia nervosa, becomes fat. Acute schizophrenia usually causes loss of weight, but in chronic forms, when the patient is on a maintenance dose of a neuroleptic, he frequently becomes overweight. Indeed, weight gain is a side effect of many psychotropic drugs, notably antidepressants and lithium; it is a common reason why female patients in particular fail to continue their medication. Especially when faced with a depressed older patient, the possibility that physical disease may be responsible for weight loss must always be borne in mind. The most extreme states of emaciation occur, without doubt, in anorexia nervosa.

It is important that weight loss be restored as soon as possible, in all psychiatric disorders. Serious loss of weight itself brings about physical and mental changes; hypothalamic and pituitary functions are disturbed; obsessional behaviour and thinking increase; and the emaciated patient becomes increasingly restless, fractious and withdrawn. Psychotherapy is ineffective at low weights, one important reason for insisting that a patient with anorexia nervosa must regain weight from the start of treatment. In depressive illness the patient who fails to return to his normal weight, in spite of appearing cheerful, has not fully recovered and is liable to relapse. Similarly with schizophrenic disorders; such patients should not be discharged from hospital until they have regained their full weight.

Therapists rarely show much concern over excessive weight gain, and often leave it to the patient to take the initiative in restricting his diet. In fact, persistent fatness is an ominous sign in female patients, implying that morale and self esteem remain low, and that neurotic problems remain unresolved. Everyone has his optimum weight and every effort should be made to achieve this. Every disease, whether psychiatric or somatic aspects predominate, should be seen in its entirety, and viewed psychosomatically.

Eating is controlled by a number of interrelated mechanisms, psychological and physical, which regulate the amount eaten and the body's energy balance, and are concerned in the sensations of hunger, appetite and satiety.

Hunger comprises variable sensations of discomfort, sometimes diffuse, sometimes localised to 'the stomach', which increase in the absence of food. Hunger begins as soon as the feeling of satiety subsides, and increases steadily between one meal and the next. For most people in western society, hunger reaches perceptible proportions only just before a meal. The urge to eat depends on the time of day, custom and external events. Absorbing and exciting activity may postpone awareness, boredom and dissatisfaction can make hunger more insistent.

A component of hunger includes a feeling of emptiness in the epigastrium. This is often accompanied by gastric contractions, felt as 'rumbling'. Nevertheless, hunger is neither delayed nor diminished by gastrectomy or bilateral vagotomy. As hunger increases, feelings of weakness, cold and dryness of the throat, sometimes salivation, and a combination of fatigue and restlessness occur. Some people develop headache or feel nausea when hungry. Many become irritable, particularly when blood sugar is low.

Appetite is an anticipatory emotional state involving mental imagery. It is usually, but not invariably, inconsistent with sadness or worry. Some people, the exceptions, eat more when they are depressed or anxious, partly for the tranquillising effect of food, and partly because of its association with pleasant sensations. Appetite is normally enhanced by hunger. It may be stimulated by the sight, taste, smell or simply the thought of a dish that is liked. It vanishes with some affective states, unfamiliarity or prejudice; the more unsophisticated a person, the more likely he is to refuse strange foods or methods of preparation.

Abnormalities of appetite are well known to occur in pregnancy; craving may occasionally give way to bulimia; aversions involve compelling and unusual distaste for foods normally enjoyed. The dulling of taste which seems to occur in pregnancy is probably a factor, but not the only one. Quirks of appetite also occur in depression, in starvation and in anorexia nervosa. Appetite, like hunger, is by no means absent or even diminished in primary anorexia nervosa. Food is feared and avoided only for its effect on weight. Patients with anorexia nervosa would eat with enjoyment if they were convinced that no weight gain would result. Some of those who indulge, pleasurably, in compulsive over-eating, do so knowing that they can vomit afterwards and thus retain little nourishment.

Palatable foods stimulate hunger and appetite; and equally, hunger makes food seem more palatable. It is palatability that induces people to continue eating.

When a patient with anorexia nervosa is struggling to control her eating, she chooses the least palatable foods and, in particular, avoids anything that is sweet. On the other hand, if she has an eating binge she is likely to choose bread and jam, chocolate or sweet biscuits. Those patients who go through a phase of compulsive shoplifting frequently steal cakes and sweets, and those tense middle-aged women who get up at night and eat compulsively always choose sweet foods.

Differential assessment of palatability is diminished with increasing hunger. Under extreme hunger the urge to eat is predominant, and nutrients become acceptable which would otherwise be discarded.

Satiety is a sensation of having had enough, with cessation of the urge to eat. It is usually accompanied by a feeling of gastric fullness. The Romans, by the use of vomitoria, were able to go on eating for hours at a time. In anorexia nervosa also, self-induced vomiting is employed by some patients, since it allows them to continue eating without putting on weight. The patient with anorexia nervosa who eats compulsively seems either not to recognise satiety, or responds to it by vomiting. On the other hand, the anxious abstainer complains of feeling full after only a few mouthfuls. Fullness, however, is not the only factor in satiety. If it were, filling the stomach with methyl-cellulose would be a more successful method of inducing the obese to eat less.

Satiety in the adult seems to involve a change or relaxation of mood, which in turn is dependent on events occurring mainly at an unconscious level. It occurs too quickly—often before the end of a meal—to allow time for metabolites to enter the blood stream and suppress hunger or set up specific humoral satiety signals. Immediate satiety may be due in part to the volume of food actually ingested.

The sensation of satiety normally inhibits eating, and is therefore considered to be more important in functional eating disorders than appetite or hunger. In the obese, eating tends to be regulated not so much by appetite and satiety as by external cues; the time, the offer or availability of food. Bruch suggests that in anorexia nervosa also, internal signals concerning eating are not perceived.

Anorexia is a negative state, an absence of appetite, of the desire to eat, despite unsatisfied energy requirements. The term 'anorexia nervosa' is misleading, since it does not necessarily involve absence of appetite. Anorexia can arise in a variety of circumstances: with pyrexia; in metabolic upsets; with gastric disorders, from alcoholic gastritis to carcinoma; in some hypothalamic tumours; and in anxiety states and depression.

HYPOTHALAMIC MECHANISMS

Nutrition, reproductive activity, temperature homeostasis, sleeping and wakefulness are among the functions of the hypothalamus. Anatomically, it comprises multiple intermingled groups of specialised neurones, each part of a complex neural system. It is not yet possible to separate hypothalamic components responsible for one process from those of another. There must be a substantial degree of overlap and involvement with each other. This is particularly apparent in anorexia nervosa where disorders of nutrition, menstruation, sleep and temperature control, libido and fertility all co-exist.

Nevertheless, it is convenient to consider the hypothalamus in terms of 'centres', each having a major influence over one or other process. Experimental work and clinical observations suggest the presence of a satiety centre in the ventromedial hypothalamus and feeding and drinking centres in the lateral hypothalamus.

Neurotransmitter control of hypothalamic functions

The various specialised neurones of the hypothalamus are served by such neurotransmitters as noradrenaline, dopamine, serotonin and acetylcholine. Noradrenaline and dopamine appear to be concerned with eating, drinking and the 'reward system'. Acetylcholine seems to be linked with cortical activation, satiety and fearfulness.

Factors affecting the eating control centres

The hypothalamic centres are influenced by cognitive, biochemical and thermal information. The first of these includes awareness by the individual of how much he has ingested.

Usually a raised blood glucose is associated with feelings of satiety. Mayer suggests that it is the rate of utilisation of glucose, rather than the level, that is significant; indicating that it is not the level of glucose alone that produces hunger. In diabetics, in whom glucose utilisation is impaired despite a high blood level, hunger is still present. Glucagon is released in response to a meal, and provides the earliest biochemical information about it to the hypothalamus, together with cholecystokinin, a hormone released from the gut.

Thermostasis

Brobeck postulated that the hypothalamus may regulate feeding behaviour in response to changes in the heat balance of the body.

Thermogenesis, produced by a rise in metabolic rate, follows the ingestion of a reasonably large meal, particularly one with a high protein content. It may be noticed part-way through the meal. Miller has proposed thermogenesis as a physiological response in people who do not grow fat despite a calorific intake much beyond their apparent energy needs.

Long-term regulation of weight

These feedback mechanisms acting upon the hypothalamic centres for nutrition seem to be effective only for short-term regulation of energy balance. Long-term regulation, often of great precision, also takes place. Wide variation of intake may occur from day to day, but compensatory changes occur automatically to restore the energy reserve held in adipose tissue over a period of a week or more. Daily weighing of a patient may be misleading, and impede his motivation and progress.

The matter of exercise is questionable. While exercise may increase appetite, there is no evidence that eating results in more exercise-taking. It is well known that the obese are less active than others. In anorexia nervosa there is usually compulsive over-activity.

ANOREXIA CAUSED BY PSYCHIATRIC DISORDER

In most depressive illnesses, especially when endogenous features are present, both hunger and appetite are lost. The depressed patient has no interest in food and, unless he forces himself to eat rapidly loses weight. If he resorts to alcohol to counteract his misery he may maintain his weight, or even increase it. Signs of vitamin deficiencies are unusual unless the condition is long standing.

In the majority of successfully treated patients appetite is regained as depression lifts, and weight soon returns to normal. Before antidepressants became available, a significant proportion of patients relapsed after appearing to improve with e.c.t. It was noticeable that most of these failed to regain their former weight. In contrast, those who continued to progress after e.c.t. quickly recovered their weight.

The use of antidepressant drugs has altered this picture in several ways. These drugs have replaced e.c.t. in milder states of depression; and are continued until depression remits naturally. Weight is recovered quickly by most patients; so much so that about 20 per cent complain of putting on an excessive amount of weight. Those patients who remain underweight, usually show other depressive symptoms, and may well benefit from e.c.t.

In the past, modified insulin was sometimes used to stimulate hunger and appetite in underweight depressives. This is rarely needed today. (See section below on Anorexia Nervosa.)

Small doses of phenothiazine derivatives will sometimes encourage a patient to eat. Chlorpromazine up to 75 mg a day, is an effective drug in relaxing tension, stimulating appetite and putting on weight, particularly in neurotic depressive states, and anorexia nervosa. When much weight has been lost the addition of an anabolic steroid is helpful. Vitamins, orally or by injection, are a sensible precaution when a patient is known to have eaten an illbalanced diet for 6 or more months.

Tube feeding is virtually never required today, except as a rare life saving necessity. Depressive and catatonic stupor and schizophrenic negativism lift quickly after e.c.t., and emaciation, however extreme, is no contra-indication. As the psychotic state lifts so the patient can be persuaded and encouraged to eat.

ANOREXIA NERVOSA

Anorexia nervosa, a rare condition a century ago, is now frequently seen. Dieting is commonplace in adolescent girls, particularly those around 16 to 18. Most of them diet reasonably, or give up after a few weeks. But about 1 per cent of intelligent schoolgirls between 16 and 18 now develop anorexia nervosa. It mainly affects girls in the upper socio-economic classes, although males can also develop the condition.

To diagnose anorexia nervosa there must be *active* refusal by the patient to eat enough to maintain weight, and/or determined efforts to prevent ingested food from being absorbed, by vomiting or the use of purgatives. There must also be amenorrhoea (although primary amenorrhoea is present in a small proportion of patients, and male anorexia nervosa poses difficulties). The age of onset of most patients (see below) lies between 11 and 35 years; although cases of atypical anorexia nervosa can develop any time after this. There must of course be no sign of organic disease which might account for weight loss, serious affective disorder, or schizophrenia.

Pattern of eating behaviour

Signs and symptoms of anorexia nervosa are liable to change and vary with the duration of the condition. All patients at the start of anorexia nervosa restrict the amount they eat, particularly starchy foods. Only around 70 per cent of them profess to diet in order to lose weight. The remainder claim that they are only able to eat small amounts because of abdominal discomfort, difficulty in swallowing, or simply because they have no sense of hunger and appetite; they deny wanting to be thin, and may even express concern over their loss of weight. These patients are likely to be older than those pursuing thinness, and to display 'atypical' features.

We believe, along with others, that there is a typical or primary form of anorexia nervosa. The patient at onset is aged between 11 and 19 years, is intelligent and attractive, and fanatically pursues thinness for its own sake. She is very active and is continually exercising, largely in order to enhance weight loss.

She may start to diet on her own, or with a group of friends, although sooner or later the latter drop out of the race. She herself may have made several ineffectual attempts to diet in the past. If she is overweight, and about 40 per cent of these primary patients are plump before anorexia nervosa, she probably diets at first with family and social approval, with a proclaimed weight target. But when this is reached, instead of then relaxing her diet, she maintains it and may even intensify it.

Weight loss may be slow but steady, progress stepwise, or be precipitous. Sooner or later the patient's increasingly emaciated appearance arouses concern among those around her. She denies, for her part, any worry. Her weight is 'just right', she still feels 'too fat', or she is not yet thin enough. The contrast between her skinny appearance, often with cyanotic extremities, and her energy and restless activity, and between the understandable concern of her parents and her own insistence that she never felt better, is striking. It is difficult for the uninitiated not to follow their instinct and seize the girl by the scruff of the neck and attempt to force her to eat a proper meal. The parents have probably already tried. Failure is almost inevitable. Few weapons are as powerful as a hunger strike.

Hunger and appetite

Hunger is not lost at first and the girl often has to battle hard against her pangs. Occasionally she lapses, but such is the sense of guilt and self-disgust afterwards that this gives her additional determination and willpower to succeed. However, as time passes and her food supply is increasingly reduced, hunger diminishes and may disappear altogether; this process can take up to a year or so.

Appetite on the other hand may increase. The girl thinks with pleasure all day long of food, particularly if she has gained control of the meal table and does not anticipate pressure to eat more than she intends. She may insist on her meals being 'perfectly' cooked and presented, minute as they are. She may eat very slowly, savouring every mouthful to the full, cutting the food into tiny pieces. Sometimes, but only after the condition has become established, she insists on cooking for herself (the only way she can be sure that her intake is right), or on eating alone. She can then enjoy the meal without feeling watched, and she is sure of giving nothing of herself away.

Appetite receives indirect satisfaction from reading cookery books and articles, studying and learning the calorific values of foodstuffs, cooking for the family, watching others eat, hoarding, and sometimes stealing food; although this is rare before the appearance of eating binges. While she herself specifically avoids fattening foods, particularly carbohydrates, she delights in cooking fattening meals for her parents, and is most upset when any food is left uneaten.

Her energy is prodigious, and she is continually engaged in physical activity, going for walks, cleaning the house, riding her bicycle. She usually denies feeling tired in the early stages, even though she may have lost 10 kg (22 lb) or more, but later on many patients admit to fatigue, that they have to force themselves to exercise when really they want only to rest. Some, however, maintain to the end that they feel 'full of energy'. Rarely, fluids are also refused, partly because dehydration abolishes hunger, but mainly because the patient believes that this will increase her loss of weight.

A few of these patients with primary anorexia nervosa continue into chronicity; 20 years later their eating behaviour and attitudes to food are the same. But for the most part, from around 9 months onwards, or even earlier, changes occur in their style of eating. Suddenly the patient finds that she has lost her self-control over eating. Eating binges now alternate with desperate attempts to re-establish dieting, but inexorably overeating gains mastery; weight therefore increases, although it may swing up and down as episodes of abstention briefly succeed bulimia. Sooner or later this depressing oscillation levels out and eating gradually becomes normal.

However a number of patients short-circuit this natural process of restitution. They learn to counteract their eating binges, and so control their weight, by vomiting. Others employ not only vomiting, but also purging, and take large quantities of laxatives after binges. Binging and vomiting is a reinforcing pattern; there is intense satisfaction from overeating, and pleasurable relief in vomiting. These patients therefore often continue this behaviour for a very long time, the more so as it is secretive, often unsuspected even by those living closest to them. Hysterical mechanisms and atypical features are particularly liable to arise in such patients. They merge imperceptibly with the atypical or secondary forms of anorexia nervosa.

Many of these patients seem to be unable to recognise when they are satiated, a feature regarded by Bruch as important for diagnosing primary anorexia nervosa. Some of the bingers eat huge quantities with no feeling of fullness; these patients often vomit afterwards. Others feel full up after a minute quantity of food. 'If only I know how much I needed to eat not to put on weight', is a common cry.

Weight

The patient with primary anorexia nervosa is terrified of fatness, and seeks thinness relentlessly. Thinness symbolises idealism, goodness, perfection, and ultimately protection and freedom from anxiety. Thinness desexualises her, irons out her developing body and abolishes libido, and allows her not to be a grown-up woman. At the same time her refusal to eat is her own choice, her assertion that she is independent, that she has no need to share anything, food or her feelings, with others.

Many adolescent girls have a distorted perception of the size of their bodies, seeing themselves as fatter than they really are, particularly around the waist, hips and thighs. This tendency is understandably exaggerated in anorexia nervosa, particularly the primary kind. They see themselves as 'fat', even when they recognise, in a moment of reality, how thin they really are. Many of these primary patients look at themselves regularly in the mirror for reassurance that they are on the right road to thinness. Some derive intense pleasure from 'mirror gazing' and spend time doing so each day; narcissism of this degree is a bad prognostic sign. But some girls, usually those who have been emaciated for 2 or more years, are upset by looking at their bodies, particularly their hips; afraid that they may find signs of fatness, and therefore signs of their own greed and lack of control.

Bruch regards 'a disturbance of delusional proportions in the body image and body concept', as being an essential symptom of primary anorexia nervosa. 'Delusional' is probably too strong a word here, since the symptom is only an exaggeration of a virtually normal trait, and many patients are able to recognise the absurdity of their claims, even though they cannot abandon the idea that their emaciated figures are still too fat. Nonetheless, even when a patient has such limited insight, this is temporarily lost as soon as she has to eat. All sense of proportion is lost if the patient has to eat a meal outside her own controlled routine. To eat with friends means that she must go without one or two of her usual meals beforehand, to have to eat at an unexpected time, e.g. midday, automatically rules out the evening meal, and causes anxiety and depression.

Patients with secondary anorexia nervosa (see Table 7.1), do not have this disturbance of body image and concept. They may proclaim that they are too fat, that they must become thinner, but this is not because they are chasing thinness for its own sake. Rather, such patients want to lose weight because of the effect this has on those who are closest to them; they lose weight in order to manipulate other people, for some much-needed although, to other people, negligible gain.

Loss of weight may be extreme in both primary and secondary cases, and even result in death; the lowest weight of any of our patients was 20·25 kg (45 lb). At very low weights oedema of the feet, and periorbital oedema, is sometimes striking. Most of the characteristic signs and symptoms of primary anorexia nervosa are the direct result of starvation

Table 7.1 Differences between primary and secondary (atypical) anorexia nervosa.

	Primary	Secondary
Usual age range	11 – 18 years	19 years +
Body image distorted	Always	Rarely
Appetite and hunger	Often strong at first, and requires much will power to resist	Often anorexic from the start
Appreciation of food	Greatly enjoyed, provided it does not lead to fear of increasing weight	Not enjoyed
Knowledge of calorific value of foodstuffs	Considerable	Often limited
Interest in cookery	Large	Often none
Menstruation	Stops with the onset of dieting. Return is delayed for many months after weight has been regained	Often stops after weight has been lost. Periods sometimes return immediately weight is regained
Sexual activity	Virtually none	Frequent. Often engaged or married
Precipitating factors	Important exams	Sexual intercourse
Activity	Always great	Often slight
Lanugo hair	Frequently seen	Rare
Bradycardia	Always at low weights	Often tachycardia
Acrocyanosis	Extreme	Variable

and emaciation; hypotension, bradycardia, hypothermia and hypersensitivity to cold, growth of lanugo hair, dry skin and head hair, acrocyanosis, carotenaemia, facial pallor, paronychia, constipation and reduced sleep. Patients with secondary anorexia nervosa may have persistent tachycardia, or this may appear only after an eating binge, lanugo hair is less likely to be present, and acrocyanosis and carotenaemia are not nearly so common.

Amenorrhoea

Amenorrhoea is essential for a diagnosis of anorexia nervosa. There are many patients with phobic anxiety and reactive depression whose weight loss is considerable, but menstruation is still present, perhaps sparse and irregular. Although some of these cases have an outward similarity to secondary anorexia nervosa, we exclude them because they lack the hypothalamo-pituitary dysfunction characteristic of anorexia nervosa.

Menstruation is closely associated with weight and changes of weight. There is a critical weight for menarche. When a patient's weight falls below her critical level menstruation is likely to stop, and only resumes when that weight has been regained. Amenorrhoea can certainly develop as a result of starvation, but loss of weight is not the cause of amenorrhoea initially in anorexia nervosa, certainly not in the vast majority, and never in primary anorexia nervosa. Menstruation stops, in most cases of primary anorexia nervosa, when the patient begins to diet. Once the patient becomes emaciated, of course, the low weight reinforces the original hypothalamic 'switch-off'.

A few patients, usually those with secondary anorexia nervosa, develop amenorrhoea up to a year or more after weight loss, but occasionally long before it. Most patients resume menstruation when they regain satisfactory weight. However, there is usually a prolonged period between restoration of weight and menstruation in primary anorexia nervosa; the average time is 9 months. Menstruation is likely to return more quickly in secondary anorexia nervosa; sometimes immediately refeeding is started, and often before the critical weight is reached.

Most patients with primary anorexia nervosa are pleased when menstruation stops, although about half want to be reassured that it will return and their fertility will not be impaired. This is part of their idealism; motherhood is seen as an ideal, unconnected with a sexual relationship. Patients with secondary anorexia nervosa are more concerned; when fear of pregnancy lies behind their refusal to eat there may be defensive overconcern about amenorrhoea. Libido is invariably lost in primary, and frequently in secondary anorexia nervosa, although when fear of pregnancy is removed, the latter may show increased libido for a time.

Most of our patients are females and the majority have already menstruated before developing anorexia nervosa. But 9 per cent have not started their periods. These female patients with primary amenorrhoea pose the same problem of diagnosis as males. Yet they present such a typical clinical picture of anorexia nervosa that is would be pedantic to exclude them. All our patients with primary amenorrhoea at onset, who have regained their normal weight, are now menstruating; the average time after recovery of weight is 2 years.

Types of treatment

In a condition of such diversity, it is understandable that a wide range of treatments has been employed. In many ways we have not improved on the methods recommended by Gull. If anorexia nervosa has been present for more than a year, or if the patient is emaciated, it is nearly always necessary to separate her from her family and bring her into hospital. It can be dangerous, particularly for the inexperienced therapist, to treat a patient with anorexia nervosa as an outpatient, since he may inadvertently allow her to procrastinate and 'play games' without any real physical or mental improvement. This reinforces the problems which exist at home between her and the rest of the family. The result may be that the therapist ends up by virtually colluding with the patient in her retreat from reality, her regression and refusal to grow up.

Primary anorexia brings emotional development to a halt, and stops both physical and psychological maturation at an important stage. This in itself is an urgent reason for insisting that a patient regains weight steadily, and enters hospital if she fails to do so. It is essential that the therapist makes this understood by the patient and her relatives from the outset. In most cases, the weight target is around 90 per cent of the ideal weight for the patient's age, sex and height. This target should be agreed upon with the patient as soon as possible.

The reasons for placing such emphasis on regaining weight from the beginning, include not only bare survival but reversal of the psychological and hormonal changes which accompany anorexia nervosa. As long as a patient remains well below her critical weight, the activity of the hypothalamo-pituitary axis is impaired. The output of pituitary gonadotrophins is diminished and the normal pattern of secretion disturbed.

The mental unrest and difficulty in concentration that characterise an emaciated patient, begin to diminish only when weight is recovered. Noticeable psychological changes occur when 80 per cent of normal weight is passed. The patient becomes more outgoing, concentrates better, is cheerful, and her interest in people and outside activities returns. At this point her preoccupation with her body size and with food and fatness lessens. She may even be able to admit that her worries about her weight are ridiculous, even though she may still feel 'too fat'. Mentally she becomes more receptive and adaptable, and it is only now that the problems and difficulties underlying her refusal to eat and loss of weight can be probed and discussed constructively.

The initial interview is included here because of its importance on treatment and its outcome. Not only is the diagnosis established, but the foundations of a psychotherapeutic relationship are laid, and a treatment plan made and agreed upon. The patient needs to feel that her fears and behaviour are understood, and that the therapist recognises her sense of helplessness. Following this she may be able to admit that she is terrified of the consequences of her refusal to eat and that she wants help in arresting the weight loss. This is an important admission, and can be used to strike a bargain. Some therapists insist on hospital admission at once. We believe, unless the patient is very emaciated, that it is better to give her the choice of putting on an agreed weight, say 2·5 kg (5 lb) in 2 weeks or, failing this, to enter hospital. The patient comes to the clinic on her first visit accompanied usually by her parents or, if married, her spouse. It is our custom to see the patient on her own first, for about 45 minutes, then her parents or husband for 20 minutes, then finally the patient and family together to discuss the plan of treatment. A bargain is struck with the patient and an acceptable weight target agreed upon in most cases. This is based upon tables of 'ideal weight', according to age and build, but also takes into account the patient's 'normal' weight.

Rapport and trust are established as a patient senses that the therapist understands her dilemma over eating. Discussion about her style of eating leads on naturally to her describing the behaviour of her parents at meal times and the struggles that ensue. This in turn results in her considering her relationships with her family and how they communicate with one another. Possible reasons why she refuses to eat, or overeats and vomits, may be touched on and explored gently at the first interview, but for most patients this is initially too threatening and may cause them to re-erect mental barriers. In any case, more knowledge about the family is needed before the psycho-dynamics of any patient with anorexia nervosa can be fully appreciated. Even then, it is important to recognise that the therapist sees only a small part of the whole.

At no time should a therapist threaten or cajole a patient. Not only does this destroy rapport, but it shows the patient that the therapist either does not understand her ambivalence about food and weight, or has no patience and no respect for her. A patient's agreement to whatever treatment is undertaken is vital, even though this may be qualified by her doubts and fears. If she refuses totally to co-operate, to agree to reach a reasonable weight, the therapist should withdraw his offer of help. Although she may express her misgivings at length, or even go away, it is rare for the patient finally to decide not to try the proposed plan.

The interview with relatives is valuable and provides a range of information. The patient and her relatives are finally seen briefly together and the plan of treatment outlined, discussed and agreed upon. The patient needs to feel that her parents are supporting and not simply abandoning her. She has to recognise that the therapist is capable of taking charge and dominating the therapeutic scene. She wants to know that he is on her side and that she can trust him.

The initial interview in some cases is enough to 'cure' the patient. Both the girl and her parents come to see her behaviour in a new light, recognise the problems which underline her symptoms, and are sufficiently secure as a family and mature enough to adapt accordingly.

Inpatient regime

Inpatient treatment depends to some extent upon whether the patient is an abstainer or a binger/vomiter.

On arrival in the ward, the procedure is explained to the patient and to any accompanying relative. The patient must remain in hospital until she reaches and retains for about 2 weeks her target weight; about 90 per cent of her ideal weight. At first the patient is on total bed-rest. She is weighed each day at the same time; immediately on rising and after emptying the bladder, but before breakfast or drinking any fluid. As her weight increases she gains privileges; she is allowed up to the lavatory, to have a bath, to use the telephone, dress and be up all day, go for a walk, spend a weekend at home and, ultimately, if she maintains her weight, leave hospital. At first she is allowed no visitors, neither family nor friends. Visiting is a privilege she must win by attaining an agreed weight.

It is often a useful incentive for a patient to have her weight chart on the wall beside her bed. Its presence also has the effect of diminishing her fear of increasing weight. Rarely a patient asks not to be told her daily weight gain. There is no point in making an issue over this; once the 80 per cent critical point is reached, a perceptive change in outlook towards weight develops, and her fears diminish. In any case the nurse weighing her each morning indicates by her approving response that she is gaining satisfactorily.

Some abstainers eat everything they are given as soon as they enter hospital. Bingers/vomiters rarely present a problem in this respect. Sometimes this reflects their resentment at being admitted and determination to leave by reaching the 'home' weight target as quickly as possible. More often it is because patients feel that they no longer have to control their appetites and can abandon themselves safely to the nursing staff.

Others are extremely difficult to persuade to eat. They may refuse point blank to co-operate, throw food on the floor or at the nurses supervising them, take tiny amounts and chew each mouthful a hundred times, or scream and weep every time they are asked to eat. But most patients, however resistant initially, eventually give in and co-operate with relief when they have satisfied themselves that the staff are capable of taking control.

Particularly if a patient is emaciated and has been literally starving herself to death, it is advisable to begin re-feeding with a bland milky diet of about 1500 calories, giving small amounts at 2-hourly intervals. To give too large or solid a diet on admission is to run the risk of paralytic ileus or acute gastric dilatation.

The amount of food is gradually increased until, after 10 to 14 days, the patient is having a diet of between 4000 and 5000 calories a day. A typical day's diet comprises:

Breakfast:	Porridge, with milk and sugar; two scrambled eggs on buttered toast; two rounds of toast; butter and marmalade; milky coffee.

Mid-morning snack:	Cereal-fortified milk drink; two rounds of toast; butter and honey or jam.
Lunch:	Normal portion of meat and green or root vegetables, with two scoops of mashed potato. Sponge pudding or pie with custard; or milk pudding.
Mid-afternoon snack:	As for the morning.
Supper:	As for lunch.
Evening snack:	As for the morning and afternoon snacks.

The emphasis is on carbohydrate: double helpings of potatoes, but not of meat. Snacks between main meals consist of cereal fortified drinks, with toast, butter and jam. Toast is readily digested, as it has already been partially converted into dextrins.

Reassurance must be given frequently, particularly to the abstainer, and especially in the first fortnight, that the patient's weight is correct, neither fat nor thin.

It is important that a patient gets into the pattern of eating all she is given from the moment she arrives in hospital. This means that, on the one hand meals must be chosen which the patient is physically capable of managing, and on the other that firm persuasion is unrelenting. Encouragement is constantly necessary.

Even the most experienced nurse can be deceived by these patients into believing that they have eaten all they have been given. The only reliable indicator that a patient is eating satisfactorily is a steady gain in weight. Some patients try to deceive by drinking a pint or more of water (bath water if given the chance), by not urinating for many hours before weighing, and of course, if they can, by concealing weights about their bodies, anything ranging from bath crystals to coins. Food may be hidden in a pillow case or between the blankets, and later transferred to bags and thrown out of the window, flushed down the wash basin or lavatory, or transferred to a collusive fellow patient. Vomiters may use plastic bags for their vomit, unless they already have access to the lavatory or basin; it is not unknown for the basins to become blocked with partially digested foodstuffs.

Weight does not necessarily increase in a steady curve. Initially there may be a dramatic increase of weight due to water retention. This is inevitably followed by a plateau when there appears to be no weight gain, or even a slight loss. Palpable abdominal tightness is an indication that intake needs to be reduced temporarily. Eating everything she is given, a patient should gain at least 1·5 kg (3·3 lb) a week.

After the first week or so, the weight chart is a remarkably sensitive indicator of a patient's emotional state and progress, as well as her degree of co-operation. For instance, a patient may regularly lose weight whenever her parents visit. Not only is this suggestive evidence of perhaps still undisclosed family tensions, but it is an occurrence which can be shown to the patient and discussed. A large fall of weight may also occur when a patient is allowed home for the weekend. This invariably indicates that she is not yet ready to cope with emotional problems at home. Again, it is important to discuss why she has lost weight. One reason why psychotherapy alone, without refeeding, is so often unproductive is that variations in weight are the patient's major method of communication in this illness. It is only when her weight approaches near normal that the patient can begin to formulate her fears and conflicts. Equally, restoration of weight without helping the patient to understand what underlies her eating behaviour, is likely to be of temporary benefit only.

Inpatient treatment of vomiters and laxative abusers. Patients who habitually control their weight by vomiting or laxative abuse are likely to be older, 19 and upwards. On admission, patients are frequently found to have disturbed plasma electrolytes. Hypokalaemia is common and care must be taken to restore this. These patients are among the most devious, and are adept at getting relatives to send them laxatives by post, or other patients to buy them. Obviously such patients require close supervision.

We rely mainly upon response-prevention for vomiters, but have occasionally employed the technique of telling the patient that she will have to eat anything she vomits. One practical demonstration is usually enough to break the pattern. All these behavioural manoeuvres are merely a preliminary to treatment of the underlying problem, which always involves a distorted relationship with a key figure or figures. In contrast to the young abstainer, it is essential from the start to focus upon what the patient is achieving by her behaviour, and in what way the other person concerned is colluding with her. It is common to find that the husband or fiancé of a patient is as terrified as she is of a full, adult relationship. Both partners escape from the real issues by concentrating on the patient's vomiting or laxative abuse.

In these cases inpatient treatment may be needed either for medical reasons or, more often, to break the habit. From the outset, while the therapist explores the problem and develops rapport with the patient, a co-therapist interviews the husband, or other close relative or friend involved in the situation. Joint interviews are later set up with the patient, partner, and the two therapists, with the aim of helping the couple to recognise each other's needs and develop better ways of communicating their feelings to one another. Ultimate success depends to a great extent on the personality strength of the partner.

Drugs in the treatment of anorexia nervosa

Chlorpromazine and other phenothiazine derivatives. Psychotropic drugs are particularly useful for patients in hospital. They reduce their anxiety and enable the patient to overcome her fear of eating. Their use in out-patients is less helpful and predictable.

Chlorpromazine is still the drug of choice, although there are theoretical objections to its use. Twenty years ago it was used in combination with 'modified' insulin; the latter was given with the purpose of increasing appetite. Today insulin is rarely used, but is discussed later. Ten years ago we gave chlorpromazine routinely to all our patients, whatever their age and mental state. In the past 7 years, only 30 per cent of patients admitted to our unit have received chlorpromazine, even briefly; these have mainly been patients in the older and middle age ranges who were restless and anxious and could not be 'persuaded' to eat by 'unending patience' on the part of the nursing staff. Although most of our patients have been persuaded to eat without the help of chlorpromazine, some have benefitted from hypnotics, anxiolytics and antidepressants.

Chlorpromazine is given by mouth, usually starting with 75 to 300 mg daily, in three or four divided doses. This can be increased if necessary to a maximum of around 1200 mg a day, according to the patient's tolerance for the drug. Caution is needed with an emaciated patient whose blood pressure is already likely to be low.

If a patient refuses to eat, chlorpromazine is given in small doses at first. The blood pressure is recorded 4-hourly for the first few days. The possible risks are small because such patients are on full bed-rest. The dosage is steadily increased every 3 or 4 days until the patient's fears and resistance are overcome and she allows herself to eat. As her anxiety diminishes, so too does the postprandial discomfort which so often reinforces her fears. If a patient resists taking chlorpromazine the drug is more easily given in the form of a syrup or suspension; the former has the disadvantage, if taken for long, of causing soreness of the tongue and mouth. Given before meals, it has the advantage of being rapidly absorbed, and producing an unpleasant numbness in the mouth which the patient is glad to remove by eating.

Side effects from chlorpromazine can be unpleasant, particularly those affecting the extrapyramidal system. Signs of Parkinsonism appear in 17 per cent of patients when 300 mg or more of chlorpromazine are given daily. Dyskinetic reactions, often involving swallowing and protusion of the tongue, develop in 8 per cent. Restlessness (akathisia) occurs in 6 per cent. These extrapyramidal effects respond to antiParkinsonian drugs and/or reduction in the dosage of chlorpromazine.

Grand mal seizures occur in around 10 per cent of patients, usually in the first fortnight of treatment, and probably result not only from the direct epileptogenic action of chlorpromazine, but also because of fluid retention. However, it is relevant to note that 25 per cent of patients requiring admission show electroencephalographic abnormalities, mostly of a non-specific kind. This proportion drops to 10 per cent in the next 3 months as weight is regained. None of our outpatients with a history of epilepsy, who gained weight slowly, had a fit, but 50 per cent of inpatients known to have epilepsy had grand mal fits, although they were not treated with chlorpromazine. This suggests that water retention, so common in the first weeks of inpatient re-feeding, is the important factor here.

The use of chlorpromazine has made it easier to treat difficult, resistant patients in hospital, and enable them to put on weight. It has been suggested that chlorpromazine is contraindicated in anorexia nervosa, because it raises prolactin levels and can cause amenorrhoea when given for long periods in high dosage. Like all phenothiazine derivatives, chlorpromazine antagonises dopamine, an inhibitor of prolactin release, but when the drug is stopped prolactin levels fall quickly to normal.

Chlorpromazine is not usually given for more than 3 or 4 weeks to inpatients, since its main value is in helping a patient to start eating. Once weight begins to increase the need for the drug diminishes. The long-term side effects of chlorpromazine do not, therefore, apply to inpatients. Chlorpromazine is occasionally useful in doses of 10 to 25 mg three times a day before meals for outpatients.

Insulin. Insulin was widely used some years ago, both on its own and in combination with chlorpromazine. The rationale for its use is that it induces unpleasant effects; sweating, dizziness, anxiety and hunger. These subside when the blood sugar rises, and so indirectly the patient is encouraged to eat; but hunger is seldom absent in anorexia nervosa, and insulin therapy is therefore not a logical approach.

Emaciated patients may be particularly sensitive because of initial high insulin levels, lack of glycogen reserve and small body mass. Insulin, even in very small dosage, is dangerous in such patients and deaths have been reported. We no longer use it.

Anxiolytics and sedatives. Benzodiazepine derivatives are often helpful in reducing the anxiety of patients sensitive to chlorpromazine, and of those who merely need sedating for the first few days of admission. A hypnotic at night is sometimes helpful, since undernourishment is associated with restless sleep. Nitrazepam can be used, although a small dose of one of the sedating tricyclic antidepressants like amitriptyline or trimipramine may induce relaxation better, especially in the older patient.

Antidepressant drugs. These may be indicated at some stage of treatment, particularly for older patients. Many of these patients are depressed in mood, although this is usually superficial and understandable, given their state and circumstances. Fifty per cent of our older patients receive an antidepressant, usually amitriptyline, during their stay in hospital, and about three-quarters continue with the drug for some time after discharge. Most cases of primary anorexia nervosa, particularly the young patients, do not require antidepressant drugs when in hospital.

The tricyclics are the most useful group of antidepressants for older patients with anorexia nervosa. When their main function is to control anxiety the dosage required is small—for instance, 10 mg of amitriptyline three times a day; too large a dose produces unpleasant side effects and does more harm than good. The monoamine oxidase inhibitors (MAOIs) have little place in anorexia nervosa, although combined antidepressant therapy with Parstelin and trimipramine does occasionally help a chronic older patient.

Other treatments

Electroconvulsive therapy. E.c.t. has been recommended by some as a routine treatment of anorexia nervosa. E.c.t. in our view should only be used as a life-saving measure, when a patient is grossly emaciated, often dehydrated, adamantly refuses to eat or drink, or persistently vomits back everything she ingests. E.c.t. must be given then, not to lift depression or improve the patient's emotional state, but as an urgent life-saving means of overcoming her resistance to eating. Inevitably e.c.t. is seen by the patient as a form of punishment. She is almost certain to have been told beforehand that if she continues not to co-operate e.c.t. will be used.

Nourishment is given immediately the patient begins to recover consciousness from e.c.t.; milk, to which is added sugar, raw eggs and powdered protein. The treatment may have to be repeated several times, daily or on alternate days; sooner or later the patient accepts that she must eat. Under these circumstances e.c.t. is an unpleasant treatment for both the patient and staff, but perhaps not as distasteful as repeated tube-feeding in a resistant patient. We have only needed to use e.c.t. in one patient with primary anorexia nervosa in the last 10 years; an incidence of less than 0·25 per cent. We have not used tube-feeding at all in the last 5 years, although in one case a nasogastric tube had to be introduced because of gastric dilatation in a purgative abuser.

Psychosurgery. Sargant was the first to report on the use of pre-frontal leucotomy as a treatment for anorexia nervosa. Since then there have been numerous reports of its use. All the published accounts are of highly obsessional patients, most of whom had severe obsessive-compulsive symptoms in addition to anorexia nervosa. The short-term effects of prefrontal leucotomy are often dramatic, and even life-saving. The patient begins to eat compulsively and put on a large amount of weight. Menstruation returns after many years' absence. But the reported follow-up periods are short.

There is no doubt that the relapse rate, after early improvement is high. Depression is also a complication and may lead to suicide. In 7 of our cases, treated by psychosurgery, 2 have been unqualified successes, 2 are partially improved, 2 are virtually unchanged, and 1 has killed herself.

Psychotherapy. Psychotherapy is a much misused and misunderstood term. We use it to describe the interactions which take place between patient and therapist on any level. It can range therefore from talk of relatively unimportant events and relationships, to discussion of her feelings for her parents, her anxieties about her family, her fears of growing up and becoming a socially and sexually mature woman, and how she deals with her resentments and unacceptable feelings.

We believe that it is necessary to be flexible in the type of psychotherapy used, as in every other aspect of treatment in anorexia nervosa. In general, it is better to concentrate on 'psychic synthesis' rather than analysis of defences. A young patient of 12 or 13 does not generally benefit from examining her psychosexual fears. Her ambivalent feelings of dependence need to be recognised and taken into consideration before members of her family are subjected to what may seem to her to be hostile criticism. The therapist should not anticipate the deep positive transference with these young patients which so frequently develops with older adolescents. The young patient with anorexia nervosa is not yet ready to separate herself from her family and stand on her own feet, to reject her mother as the model of adult womanhood, and proclaim her own separate identity. On the other hand, this may be precisely what the therapist is aiming to achieve with the older patient. For such a patient to separate herself satisfactorily, she must depend for some time on her therapist. In contrast to younger patients, prolonged follow-up treatment for a year or more is essential for most of these older patients.

Psychotherapy with one or both parents, or husband, is usually an important adjunct. The parent's role rapidly becomes that of patient, as his or her characteristics, needs and expectations are explored. Again care has to be taken over such exploration, and the vulnerability of many of the parents of patients must be recognised and accepted from the start. Otherwise a parent is liable to become unco-operative as his worst fears and anxieties are too quickly realised.

The therapist dealing with the parents should not ideally be directly involved with the treatment of the patient. He must recognise that the latter's behaviour may stem from long-standing parental disharmony. A marriage may be on the verge of breaking up, held tenuously together by the illness of the patient.

Marital relationships are particularly likely to be strained with young patients. Their parents are frequently depressed and demoralised. A depressed mother retreats from the demands and pressures of her teenage children and often creates a sense of rejection. Faced with a young patient still intensely dependent on a depressed mother, it is essential to treat the latter. Mother, with or without father, must become the main target of treatment for the child to recover and resume a natural development.

If the patient is married at the start of anorexia nervosa, she has already transferred her adolescent conflicts and problems onto her husband and has, in a sense, put some distance between herself and her family. The husband is expected to be a superman: strong, protective, understanding, loving and undemanding, thinking always of his wife and her needs. Since the type of man these immature girls choose to marry is usually himself sexually immature, wanting a woman he can look after and who does not threaten his frail masculinity, it is obvious that problems are likely sooner or later to arise. The girl finds that her needs and outlets for development are as blocked in marriage as they were with her parents. She is unable to communicate her deeper feelings to her husband. Unable to develop a more mature relationship, she protects herself and her new marital state by starvation and emaciation.

It is best to see wife and husband together, to encourage discussion of previously unacceptable topics, feelings and needs, to point out the child-like manipulation of each partner by the other. Just as parents may break up as their child improves, so also a neurotic marriage may flounder as the patient recovers and recognises the failings of her husband. At best, the crisis of anorexia nervosa upsets entrenched viewpoints so that new growth and development by both partners is possible.

Nursing problems

Nursing a patient with anorexia nervosa is extremely wearing and tests to the utmost the understanding and emotional stability of the nurse. Since 50 per cent of our student nurses, like others of their age, are themselves concerned with slimness, it is not surprising if they identify with these patients and allow themselves to be manipulated. Alternatively they may over-react and adopt an unnecessarily harsh attitude.

On admission to the ward the patient is immediately put to bed. It is the nurse who can reassure her, deal with and allay her distress, and explain once again the 'anorexic regime': the system of target and reward. It is the nurse who must usually reassure parents or other relatives who have accompanied the patient to the ward, again explaining the procedure to them and why relatives are not initially allowed to visit.

Many of the younger patients are tearful and miserable, feeling abandoned and alone. It is at this point that a nurse can do so much good, take over the role of mother to the patient, reduce her fear of putting on weight and make her feel that she is in safe hands. She must establish whether the patients has brought any food or drugs with her and tactfully take charge of these.

Since it is important to start re-feeding as soon as the patient has settled into bed, it is usually wise for an experienced nurse to bring the patient her first small meal and to remain with her. Until she has gained sufficient weight to be allowed up, a nurse has to sit with the patient during each meal. As far as possible this should be the same nurse, who will then get to know the patient and develop a mutual understanding.

If a patient reacts aggressively by throwing food away or regurgitating the nurse picks up the remains and asks the patient to eat them or, if this is impracticable, obtains fresh supplies. The strain this imposes on the nursing staff is considerable, and it is essential that they are given adequate support. No doctor can manage any but the mildest cases of anorexia nervosa without devoted co-operation from the whole of his team.

OBESITY

There are many causes of obesity; social and family, metabolic, constitutional, and psychological. Although it might seem obvious that psychological factors must invariably play a role in most cases of obesity—after all, the fat person has only to eat consistently below her energy requirements to lose weight—yet psychiatrists have failed to contribute significantly to effective treatment. The knowledge that fat people eat when bored, anxious or angry, that they derive more comfort from eating than any other activity, that eating brings back that happy association with a loving providing mother, does little to arrest a patient's nibbling or binges. Behaviour therapy can help the highly motivated, but under these circumstances, so can most treatments. Drugs provide little in the way of help.

Nevertheless, psychiatrists are often called on to deal with fatness and to investigate its psychological causes. Psychiatrists themselves often bring about undue weight gain through the drugs they prescribe. Lithium, tricyclic antidepressants, and chlorpromazine, are among the worst offenders. Many schizophrenics are unnecessarily overweight because of their maintenance drugs, which presumably affect weight and eating control centres in the hypothalamus, but any of the psychotropic drugs are liable to induce weight gain, although diazepine derivatives are unlikely to produce the gross changes that lithium and chlorpromazine may do. Occasionally treatment with a MAOI results in a patient losing weight, but this is unusual. Stopping or reducing the drug incriminated nearly always leads to loss of weight; indeed some patients refuse to continue treatment for this reason. There are obvious dangers in this for patients with schizophrenia and recurrent depression. Chlorpromazine can be replaced by a piperazine phenothiazine which, together with dietary measures, may bring about some weight loss. Lithium carbonate does not have a satisfactory substitute, although a change from a short to a long-acting form occasionally helps. For the most part, simply advising a patient to cut down on his diet achieves little.

The majority of patients who are depressed lose weight, but some gain when depressed. Such patients generally have neurotic or reactive depressions, arising from long-standing frustrations and circumstances. Women are more likely to be affected this way; their sleep is often increased sometimes to 14 or more hours a day, and at times the condition resembles narcolepsy. These patients tend to be sluggish and take little exercise; the smallest exertion results in a sense of extreme exhaustion. They usually respond well to an antidepressant, particularly a MAOI such as tranylcypromine. As symptoms lift, weight returns to normal, provided dietary advice is followed.

Bouts of compulsive eating, particularly at night (the night eating syndrome), develop in chronically tense, married, middle-aged women, with the advent of depression. They are likely to have hysterical personalities, and most of them regard their marriages as sexually unfulfilling. Their tension and depression usually respond well to a combination of an antidepressant and tranquilliser. It is more difficult to deal satisfactorily with the marital difficulties, and by no means every spouse is willing to cooperate. At the same time the patient needs to be encouraged to develop wider interests and activities, away from the narrow confines of her family.

We discussed earlier the compulsive binging that sometimes succeeds anorexia nervosa. Unless associated with vomiting, overeating invariably results in increasing weight: this is sometimes considerable. These patients have a low self esteem, and the slightest upset to their precarious equilibrium is liable to set off a bout of compulsive binging; often followed by a day or so of total starvation. This makes for even greater disruption of eating and loss of self confidence. They are nearly all in their late teens and early twenties. Understandably they become increasingly anxious and depressed, and reluctant to face their friends. As so often with psychiatric syndromes, a vicious circle arises; the more a patient withdraws into herself and relies on her own resources, the more prone she is to be overwhelmed by her appetite.

Treatment is difficult and prolonged, and calls for considerable understanding on the therapist's part. Small doses of a tricyclic antidepressant help to reduce tension. When binging is particularly bad an anorectic drug such as diethylpropion reduces hunger and appetite sufficiently to allow the patient to regain control, aided also by its mildly euphoric effect. Diethylpropion should be given for short spells only, a month or so at a time, as dependence must be guarded against.

A combined psychotherapeutic and behavioural approach is also required. The patient must eat regular small meals, learn to chew food slowly and methodically, keep a diary in which she records her eating behaviour, and any events which may have triggered off a binge. Above all she needs to feel liked and accepted by her therapist, and encouraged by his comments and optimism; or by the members of a group, such as Weight Watchers.

At times the psychiatrist may be called on to probe into the psychological problems of a seriously obese patient (without overt psychiatric symptoms), or to take over treatment. A grossly fat patient nearly always needs to be dieted in hospital at the beginning of treatment, with the aim of losing at least 10 kg (22 lb); it is important that a weight target be agreed upon by doctor and patient from the start. The patient's craving to eat can be controlled by strict bed-rest at first, with small doses of chlorpromazine. Psychological problems can be explored gently, background difficulties assessed, and a plan of behaviour evolved for when the patient returns home.

In many patients fatness is undoubtedly a protection, enabling a patient to feel more secure so far as her neurotic anxieties are concerned. When a patient diets successfully and loses much weight, depression, fatigue, headache, anxiety and other psychiatric symptoms frequently appear. She may feel incapable of readjusting to being of normal weight. Agoraphobic symptoms may have developed along with obesity, which call for treatment in their own right. Husbands may have difficulty in accepting a slim and now attractive outgoing wife. Sexual problems may arise. The psychiatrist must anticipate and deal with all these complications if his patient is to overcome obesity and remain a normal weight.

FURTHER READING

Bliss, B.P. 1973. The surgical management of obesity. *Brit. J. Hosp. Med.* July. 19.
Dally, P., Gomez, J., Isaacs, A. 1979. *Anorexia Nervosa.* Wm. Heinemann. London.
Stunkard, A. 1972. New therapies for the eating disorders. *Archives of Gen. Psychiat.* **26**. 391.

8

Treatment of sexual dysfunction and deviation

Sexual problems are extremely common in both sexes. Today, with the use of behaviour therapy, psychotherapy, and the careful use of drugs, much can be done to alleviate them. A man may complain of premature ejaculation or erectile impotence for as long as he can remember (primary), or of difficulties developing after a period of reasonably competent sexual activity (secondary). More rarely, he has no trouble with erection, but has difficulty in ejaculating in coitus; and, very infrequently, during masturbation. Both men and women may come to feel dissatisfied with what they see as a low level of sexual drive in themselves and/or their partners.

Women may complain of vaginismus, or of inability to reach orgasm. Orgasm may be possible, for example, with one partner but not with another, or in masturbation but not in coitus, or in one situation and not another.

The nature of the presenting symptom must be explored in considerable detail. It is also important to carry out a full physical examination, including appropriate laboratory investigations, to exclude physical disease such as diabetes mellitus and endocrine disorders which, if present, might be responsible for sexual dysfunction. Needless to say, no organic disease can be found in the vast majority of these patients. Recent medication with hypotensive or antidepressant drugs must be enquired about, for their side effects may include sexual difficulties. Alcohol consumption must be known, and its effect on the patient's sexual life assessed.

When no physical cause emerges, the search can move to where the trouble is most likely to lie; the nature of the patient's sexual relationship(s). He or she may be surprised at this shift of interest, and resist the implication of a partner in a matter which, up to now, they have regarded as their own problem.

An interview with the partner is of great importance, not only to learn his or her view of the sexual difficulties, but to assess the patient's motivation, and gain his co-operation for the therapeutic efforts ahead. This is then followed by joint sessions, with both partners and therapist. In the simplest cases explanation and reassurance from the therapist is enough.

The work of Masters and Johnson is too well known to bear repetition. It has had considerable influence on the way therapists think, and on the shape of therapy. Its original elements included highly motivated couples, mostly paying sizeable sums for treatment in a holiday atmosphere, and the exploration, with a male and female therapist, of their sexual relationship and values. High success rates were reported by Masters and Johnson. These were claimed to depend on the information imparted, as well as the correction of misinformation, desensitisation in vivo to the anxieties surrounding sexual intercourse, an increased awareness of sexual pleasure, and a few specific techniques. But most of all to the improved communication which developed between each of the partners.

Whether one therapist rather than the more costly two is as successful has been since questioned, and most clinics report favourable results from some modification of the methods recommended, though they are rarely as good as those of the innovators.

Two important advances since that initial work are discernible. The first concerns the orgasmic training of the dysfunctional woman, and the second focusses not only on the reduction of sexual anxieties but on the heightening of sexual arousal. In orgasmic training, women move from visual and tactile exploration of their genitals to self-stimulation, with a vibrator if necessary. In so doing they desensitise themselves to the former anxiety aroused by strong sexual excitement. They are encouraged, in relaxed circumstances, to enact the disinhibited behaviour they fear during loss of control in orgasm. This enactment is at first alone, and then with a trusted understanding partner. Some problems are more complex, for example, the partnership of a man who ejaculates prematurely and a woman unable to achieve orgasm; but the difficulties can be tackled one step at a time.

Sexual arousal may be increased by the use of fantasy or by slides, photographs and films. If part of the problem is that one partner is less appealing to the other than the fantasy or visual material, an attempt is made to switch to him or her in the seconds before orgasm. The objective is to pair the orgasmic response to the real life stimulus partner so that a classical conditioning link is established.

Most sexual therapists speak little about the relationship of the couple to the therapist. Yet the momentum of therapy depends to a large extent on how the therapist is seen; his understanding, knowledge and competence, his trustworthiness and detachment; how much each partner likes him.

Medication plays only a small part in most sexual therapy. Testosterone is still given to impotent men, but unless their own source of androgens is deficient, any effect is a placebo one. Female libido is enhanced by testosterone, and a small dose can sometimes help a sexually unresponsive woman. There is no drug that consistently increases sexual drive; i.e. is an effective aphrodisiac. Most drugs, including alcohol, which arouse desire, do so by reducing inhibitions and producing a pleasant sense of relaxation. Marihuana does just this, and allows the normally inhibited smoker to accept his sexual feelings and put them into practice, without loss of potency. Tranquillisers have their place when anxiety is prominent. Their main use lies in breaking a vicious circle of fear and failure. Anxiety at the prospect of intercourse, of yet another failure, can be reduced by one of the diazepine derivatives. But a small dose of a barbiturate, quinalbarbitone 50 mg, is sometimes more effective, particularly in highly obsessional men and women. Too much sedation will of course reduce sexual desire and defeat the purpose of treatment. When depression is present it requires appropriate treatment. And as depression lifts, so the need for specific sexual therapy may disappear. However, it is important to recognise that many of the antidepressants themselves are liable to upset sexual functions in both men and women. The MAOI may make ejaculation virtually impossible, or if it does occur it is without feeling.

The man or woman with no sexual partner poses special therapeutic difficulties. If social skills, relating for example to dating, are deficient, these can be remedied in training sessions, individually or in groups. The patient may find himself in the position of being asked by the therapist to acquire a sexual partner. But it is by no means easy to find a partner simply and solely for sexual therapy. Some clinics have found an answer in the use of surrogates. Masters and Johnson used volunteer professional women for their sexually inadequate men, in an attempt to bypass the difficulties associated with the use of prostitutes. In a survey in the United States, a high proportion of sexual therapists admitted to having had intercourse with one or more of their patients. No doubt, for some, this was the exploitation for personal gratification of their privileged position as therapists. In others perhaps, the desire to give a valuable sexual experience not otherwise available to their patient was more altruistic. But whatever the reasoning, the distortion of the relationship that must occur can only, in the long run, be disadvantageous to both patient and therapist.

SEXUAL DEVIATION

In sexual deviations—which may occur in both sexes, although those that attract society's disapproval are seen predominantly in men—unusual objects and activities cause sexual arousal. Deviations may coexist with or replace more normal and acceptable sexual activity. In exhibitionism, transvestism, paedophilia, severe sado-masochism, gerontophilia, and fetishism, a mixture of unusual object choice and activity can be seen. A partner may be involved, sometimes non-consenting.

The motivation to give up a sexual deviation may spring from fear and self-disgust, pressure from the patient's family and friends, or from society. Its strength must be assessed carefully before embarking on what may be a major therapeutic effort. The therapist must also know how the condition began and developed, although frequently the deviant can recall traces in his earliest memories, the factors that precipitate and maintain it, together with any normal sexual activity. A diary of sexual thoughts and feelings, in the period before therapy starts, may be helpful. Fantasies, impulses and actions, deviant and non-deviant, are charted. Objectives, however limited, need to be agreed on with the patient. The transvestite may accept, not to abandon transvestism altogether, but never to cross-dress at home. The heterosexual paedophile may decide to avoid future arrest by raising the age of the girls he approaches.

Therapy is directed towards:

1. Increasing a patient's self control
2. Lessening the attractiveness of the deviant sexual object or activity, and
3. Increasing the desirability of more normal sexual behaviour.

Self-control involves recognising the sequence of events that leads the patient to deviant activity, and learning how to interrupt this pattern. The transvestite comes to acknowledge that when he is alone in his flat, cross-dressing in his wife's underwear is likely to follow in the next hour. The paedophile recognises that he is child-hunting by the route he is taking and the time of day. The earlier in the sequence the patient is able to recognise what he is about, the easier it is to substitute activities incompatible with the deviance. The closer to fulfilment of his deviant need, the less capable he is of avoidance.

The patient can be electrically averted from the object or activity he wants to discard. Shocks need not be painful and can be combined with fantasy, or with real life objects and activities. The exhibitionist may shock himself, by means of a small portable apparatus, when he encounters the type of woman to whom he previously displayed his genitals.

The deviant, however, cannot be simply left desexualised by aversive techniques. The attractiveness of more normal sexuality needs to be enhanced. Fear of a partner may need desensitisation. Social skills, if deficient, must be learnt. Erectile conditioning may be engineered by pairing a vibrator stimulus (of 80 cycles per second, at the base of the penile corona) with images or slides of decreasingly deviant stimuli. Images, photographs or slides of more normal stimuli are shown, at first just before orgasm, then at increasingly longer intervals before climax.

The results of therapy, even in highly motivated sexual deviants, are understandably not as good as those achieved in sexual dysfunction. The relationship between therapist and patient is, as elsewhere, of vital importance to the patient's persistence with treatment and its outcome. Much depends on the length and quality of follow-up treatment. When behaviour therapy fails, and the sexual deviation is of an antisocial nature, the best solution may be a pharmacological one, aimed at significantly lessening the patient's sexual drive.

Oestrogens reduce male libido, although large doses, up to 15 mg a day of stilboestrol, may be required. It is advisable to start with a small dose, say 2 mg a day, and work up to an effective amount. Very high doses, given for more than a few months, result in gynaecomastia, and occasionally sterility.

Benperidol, 0·25 to 1·5 mg a day, also reduces sexual drive. Like its analogue, haloperiodol, it may cause drowsiness and extrapyramidal side effects. Cyproterone acetate is an anti-androgen and reduces the concentration of testosterone in the plasma. It has been used in the treatment of sexual offenders (who agree to its use), and has been found to reduce effectively their libido. This drug can also cause gynaecomastia, and its prolonged use may cause irreversible atrophy of the testicles.

FURTHER READING

Bancroft, J.H.J. 1974. *Deviant Sexual Behaviour: Modification and Assessment*. Clarendon Press. Oxford.

Crown, S. 1976. Marital breakdown: epidemiology and psychotherapy. In *Recent Advances in Clinical Psychiatry*. No. 2. Ed. Granville-Grossman, K. Churchill Livingstone. Edinburgh.

Heiman, J., LoPiccolo L., LoPiccolo, J. 1976. *Becoming Orgasmic: A Sexual Growth Program for Women*. Englewood Cliffs. New Jersey.

Jacobson, N.S. 1978. Marital problems. In *Symposium on Behaviour Therapy in Psychiatry*. The Psychiatric Clinics of North America. W.B. Saunders. Philadelphia.

Kaplan, H.S. 1974. *The New Sex Therapies*. Brunner/Mazel. New York.

Marks, I.M. 1976. Management of sexual disorders. In *Handbook of Behaviour Modification*. Ed. Lightenberg, H. Prentice-Hall. Englewood Cliffs, New Jersey.

McKay, D. 1976. *Psychosexual Problems: Psychotherapy, Counselling and Behaviour Modification*. Ed. Crown, S. Academic Press. London.

9

Psychiatric disorders in women

Attempts to relate female psychiatric disorders to hormonal changes have not been particularly successful. The fact that women are more likely than men to develop neurotic states can be better understood in terms of their social difficulties, and their upbringing, rather than hormone imbalance. Premenstrual tension has been elevated to what amounts almost to a mystique. Anything, it seems, from depression and anxiety to shoplifting and aggressive behaviour, is liable to envelop premenstrual woman; looked at biologically, such associations seem to be highly suspect. Schizophrenia and manic depression are shared equally between the sexes. Of the more disabling psychiatric states, unipolar depression, anorexia nervosa and agoraphobia are commoner in women.

Understandably, attention has been concentrated on pregnancy and the puerperium. A postnatal psychosis is a dramatic event, and the fact that there is almost invariably a clear period of 3 or more days after delivery before psychotic behaviour develops, and that the patient is sometimes confused at first, does suggest an organic cause, as yet unrecognised. But even here hormonal changes probably only act as triggering mechanisms, bringing a condition which was hidden but already shaped to the surface. The only factors known to be significant in the development of a postnatal psychosis are a previous episode of psychotic illness and a family history of psychosis.

Once the patient is fully orientated, the diagnosis, whether schizophrenic or affective, can be established without much difficulty. Initially the mother needs to be treated in hospital, and not separated from her baby; although measures to protect the baby may be needed if there is any risk of infanticide, or she is still delirious and incapable of feeding and caring for the child. Breastfeeding is best avoided, but there is no need to be dogmatic over this. The outlook, course and treatment of the illness are not essentially different from those of any other psychotic state.

Antidepressant drugs are begun at once when the psychosis is depressive, together with e.c.t. if depression is severe; or if confusion persists for more than a week. Mania is .best controlled by haloperidol and/or chlorpromazine, although lithium may be indicated when mania is prolonged or recurs. Schizophrenia calls for suitable doses of a phenothiazine. Once symptoms begin to lift, the patient is encouraged to take charge of the baby and assume increasing responsibility for its well being. Problems at home may need to be dealt with, and support given to the patient's family.

When a woman who has already had a psychotic illness, whether or not after childbirth, becomes pregnant the risk of a further breakdown in the puerperium is considerable; it rises from about 1 in 600 in the general population to around 1 in 6. If the patient has conceived inadvertently there are grounds for considering termination. The risk of breakdown after termination in the early stages of pregnancy is comparatively low. However, if the woman wishes to have the child, then precautions must be taken to minimise the risk.

Pregnancy itself is a safe time; it is extremely rare for serious depression or psychotic states to develop then, or for pre-existing psychoses to be exacerbated. If they do then almost certainly the patient has strongly mixed feelings over the pregnancy, and resentments towards her husband, which need to be explored.

Let us suppose our patient is a young woman who has had a depressive psychosis after her first child, which cleared up with treatment over some 6 months. Both she and her husband are keen to have another child, and have accepted the risks involved. Apart from early morning nausea in the first trimester, she has felt extremely well throughout the pregnancy and has taken no drugs.

She should have the child if possible in hospital. Psychotic symptoms developed a week after her *first* delivery. This is the critical time when she must now be carefully observed, and action taken at the first sign of abnormal thinking and behaviour. But precautions are in any case taken immediately after delivery. An antidepressant drug, preferably the one to which she responded best last time, is started as soon as she returns from the delivery room; say 75 mg amitriptyline at bedtime, and 10 mg t.d.s. Unless she has a strong preference for breastfeeding, she should not begin. This allows her greater rest at night. It also avoids the baby ingesting the antidepressant; concentration of the drug in breast milk is around one third the concentration in the mother's plasma.

A good night's sleep is important, and if necessary a hypnotic, such as flurazepam, must be given. The patient should be seen daily; any uncalled for anxiety or worrying about the baby or her husband is an indication to raise the dose of amitriptyline to 150 mg a day, and perhaps add a small dose of a neuroleptic; thioridazine 25 mg or trifluoperazine 2 mg, both three times a day. This dosage is maintained for a few days until symptoms disappear. It can then be slowly reduced, but not entirely stopped until the patient has been symptom-free for at least a fortnight.

Unless symptoms are not satisfactorily controlled by these means, and provided home conditions are reasonable, the patient can return home after a fortnight, continue her treatment there and be followed up as an outpatient. Back-up support and surveillance of the patient at home by a health visitor or district nurse, or a social worker, is important in the early weeks. She will probably need to continue the antidepressant for 6 months, the length of time of the last illness, but this must depend on the therapist's assessment of progress.

If no warning signs appear the patient can be allowed home after 9 or 10 days, provided she is seen at least weekly for the first month. The dosage of drugs can be progressively reduced and stopped, but care should be exercised for 6 months. The antidepressant should be restarted without fail if any symptoms appear during this time, however trivial they may seem. It is better to be overcautious than allow symptoms to develop insidiously and then have to deal with an established illness. Treatment in a psychiatric unit or hospital is only needed if psychiatric symptoms continue in spite of treatment. Mother and baby should be admitted together.

If psychotic symptoms developed 3 or 4 days after the first delivery, it may be advisable for the antidepressant drug to be started during the last week of pregnancy, because of the long latent period of the drug; a smallish dose, 75 mg amitriptyline, which will not affect the child significantly. Immediately after delivery the dosage is raised to 100 to 150 mg a day. Such means are called for when the risk is high, after say two previous breakdowns.

Similar precautions are taken with schizophrenic illnesses. A phenothiazine is given immediately after delivery or in the week before term. Or, if the patient is a chronic schizophrenic and has continued on a phenothiazine throughout pregnancy, it may be advisable to step up the dosage for a short time.

Postnatal blues are commonplace, and of no particular significance. They rapidly disappear for the most part with reassurance. But postnatal neurotic states, which develop some months after delivery, are a different matter. Mixtures of phobic anxiety, depression of mood, exhaustion and irritability appear and sometimes continue for years. A woman previously capable and outgoing is transformed within a short time into someone unable to cope adequately with her family responsibilities. It is the woman with a tense obsessional personality, previously able to cover up her sense of insecurity by her achievements and ability to control her world, who is liable to develop such symptoms. She may well have complained of premenstrual tension in the past and been overpossessive of her husband. All these traits are now magnified. Marital tensions develop, and the husband may react to his wife's irritability and misery by leaving her, or involving himself with another woman. Anxiety and resentment may build up to such a height that the woman may eventually collapse and require admission.

Although these postnatal neurotic states arise out of the woman's inability to adapt to her new role, psychotherapy alone is usually of small help. Symptoms respond to antidepressant medication, but particularly to a MAOI combined with a tranquilliser, say phenelzine 15 mg and diazepam 5 mg three times a day. When depressive symptoms are present, and especially when early morning waking is prominent, often the case when symptoms have been allowed to drag on for some years, combining tranylcypromine with trimipramine can bring about a dramatic improvement. Once the patient's mood and energy have improved, a combined psychotherapeutic and behavioural approach is now most helpful. Drugs may need to be continued for 6 months or more, and occasionally for several years depending upon the patient's ability to adapt, her husband's attitude, and home circumstances.

The majority of these conditions develop after the first child, and without treatment worsen with subsequent births. But occasionally a woman develops neurotic symptoms only after a third or fourth child; perhaps preceded by miscarriages. In such cases it often seems that the patient cannot adapt to the end of childbearing days; invariably there are profound problems in the marriage. Once symptoms have been lifted by suitable antidepressant treatment, marital therapy, with the couple alone or in a group, may be considered.

We have already indicated that pregnancy itself is a 'protected' period. Apart from nausea in the first 3 months many women, including not a few of those with tense insecure personalities liable to develop puerperal neurotic states later, maintain they 'never felt better'. They feel fulfilled and complete when pregnant. It is the egocentric woman with strong hysterical traits who is liable to feel tired and ill for most of her pregnancy, and occasionally may be sick throughout the 9 months. Transient minor anxieties, usually concerning the baby's normality, or risks to the patient's health, are felt by many women in the second and third trimesters, and usually respond readily to sensible reassurance.

Concern is frequently expressed about dangers to the fetus from drugs taken during pregnancy; and also while breastfeeding. Naturally, in the ideal pregnancy, no drugs should be taken, and that includes nicotine and alcohol; but in spite of recurring alarms, and some animal species, such as rats, producing abnormal offspring when given large amounts of psychotropic drugs in pregnancy, there is no firm evidence that such substances, in proper dosage, adversely affect the human fetus. *Lithium* readily crosses the placenta, and fetal lithium plasma concentration mirrors maternal levels, but many manic depressives continue lithium medication during pregnancy (see p. 29). Care must be taken to reduce lithium just before delivery, not only to ensure that the fetal lithium level is relatively low, but that the mother does not suddenly develop lithium toxicity, due to her renal clearance rate dropping after delivery. Lithium readily enters breast milk. Very occasionally the effect of a high concentration of lithium is evident in the neonate; he is hypotonic and cyanosed. These signs disappear within 48 hours.

Phenothiazines and antidepressant drugs cross the placenta, although foetal plasma concentrations are well below the maternal. However, there are a few reports of infants showing withdrawal symptoms when a mother has taken a tricyclic antidepressant throughout pregnancy.

Barbiturates and diazepine derivatives have been incriminated. A mother dependent on barbiturates may have a deformed child, and withdrawal effects need to be anticipated. Diazepam has been associated with hare lip and cleft palate; but the evidence for this is largely anecdotal. Amphetamine can cause abnormalities in rodents, but has never been shown to be teratogenic in humans. Of course, a drug's effect on the foetus may be hidden, and not apparent for many years, if at all. Progesterone, for instance, as a result of its androgenic metabolites, may induce pseudohermaphroditism, and influence developing psychosexual attitudes and functions.

Large amounts of any drug are probably capable of retarding growth, and can have an adverse effect on the neonate's functioning at birth. Babies born to alcoholic women, who continue to drink heavily throughout pregnancy, tend to be small and have an increased risk of congenital abnormalities. Withdrawal effects have been reported in the child after delivery. Any woman seeking treatment during pregnancy can be safely dried out, without affecting the baby. However, disulphuram should not be given, as this drug has been reported to cause malformations. Women addicted to opiates are liable to have babies who show typical withdrawal effects after delivery. The infants need to be carefully nursed in hospital for at least a fortnight.

We have already expressed our views on premenstrual tension and its disorders. Nonetheless, we recognise that there is a premenstrual exacerbation of symptoms in most states of anxiety and reactive depression. Indeed this is a useful differentiating pointer between reactive and endogenous depression.

Misapprehension and mistreatment of premenstrual tension abounds. A few women retain water and put on weight before periods, but this does not happen in the majority of cases. However, not a few women who complain of premenstrual tension are treated with diuretics, and become psychologically dependent on them. Although no consistent hormonal imbalance has been found with premenstrual tension, progesterone deficiency in the second half of the menstrual cycle is still claimed to exist, and exaggerated reports of successful treatment with progestational agents made. Bromocriptine has been advocated, on the grounds that prolactin is increased at this time. A variety of drugs, including lithium and most psychotropic drugs, have been advocated from time to time, with no consistently good effects.

Clearly, if water retention does accompany premenstrual tension, it is reasonable to try the effect of a diuretic. It may be reasonable to use dydrogesterone 10 mg twice a day during the premenstrual week, or a tranquilliser, always keeping an open mind and allowing for the placebo effect of such non-specific treatments. But above all the therapist must recognise that premenstrual tension is an expression of a much wider psychiatric problem.

Sooner or later, with age, menstruation stops. Once again, there is no reliable evidence that psychological disturbances arising during the menopause are related to hormonal changes. Hormonal replacement therapy is recommended by some as a cure for all menopausal miseries. Some women undoubtedly do feel better on Premarin, but on closer inspection this is because the hormone relieves unpleasant physical symptoms, such as hot sweats and flushing. Psychological factors, the end of childbearing, children leaving home, marital infidelity, fear of loss of attractiveness and desirability, lack of stimulation and outlets, probably play the major role in menopausal disturbances.

States of neurotic depression are common, and respond well to small doses of an antidepressant, followed by discussion and pinpointing of the patient's problems. Manic depression and unipolar depression sometimes develop for the first time at this period, and call for the measures already described (p. 26). Paranoid schizophrenic states begin to increase, especially among women. Alcoholism becomes an increasing problem as tolerance fails and the last vestiges of control over drinking are lost. These conditions call for energetic and skilled treatment.

FURTHER READING

Gelder, M. 1978. Hormones and post partum depression. In *Mental Illness in Pregnancy and the Puerperium*. Ed. Sandler, M. Oxford University Press. Oxford.

Granville-Grossman, K. 1971. Postpartum psychiatric problems. In *Recent Advances in Clinical Psychiatry*. Churchill Livinstone. Edinburgh.

Kendell, R.E. 1978. Childbirth as an aetiological agent. In *Mental Illness in Pregnancy and the Puerperium*. Ed. Sandler, M. Oxford University Press. Oxford.

Parlee, M.B. 1973. The premenstrual syndrome. *Psychological Bulletin*. **80**. 454.

Pitt, B. 1973. Maternity blues. *Brit. J. Psychiat*. **122**. 431.

10

Psychiatric disorders in old age

Old age, for most people, calls for considerable readjustments. Those who lack the necessary resources of personality, who become socially isolated, or whose mental functions are already in serious decline, are unable to adapt satisfactorily. The personality shifts towards introversion, hypochondriacal concern develops, and anxiety and depression may become severe enough to interfere with everyday life. Signs of dementia are liable to appear, and eventually to dominate the scene. Memory declines, judgment fails, and the old person becomes increasingly child-like in his reactions to events. Little can be done to arrest the progression of dementia, although much can be done to alleviate its consequences, not only to the patient, but also to those involved in his life. On the other hand, functional disorders respond well to psychotropic drugs and an understanding approach to the old person's problems.

The principles which lie behind the prescribing of drugs and other physical treatments to the old are no different than for young people. But it is vitally important for the therapist to recognise that renal clearance declines with age, and that a drug and its metabolites will therefore be eliminated comparatively slowly. One of our patients, who was first prescribed lithium carbonate for manic depression 24 years ago at the age of 56, then required 1200 mg a day to maintain a serum concentration of 0·8 mmol/l; today she needs a daily dose of 800 mg. The rate at which a drug is metabolised by liver enzymes is also diminished, so that the half-life of a drug is likely to be prolonged. And perhaps most important of all, the side effects of drugs are much greater in old people; hypotension, hypothermia, confusional states, unexpected outbursts of irritability, are all liable to develop from careless prescribing. There is no doubt that some old people are overdrugged, and lose many of their symptoms when drugs are withdrawn, but that is no reason for the therapist to shirk treating his elderly patients, or to prescribe in a half-hearted, inadequate manner.

Depression is common, and frequently colours anxiety and hypochondriasis in old age; it is the main reason for a patient's referral to a psychiatrist. Most cases of depression are reactive, the result of bereavement, social isolation, or other adverse circumstances, or reflect long-standing neurotic difficulties. Sometimes they occur in the setting of physical illness, and it is as well to be on guard for an undetected carcinoma, or a rare case of pernicious anaemia.

Not infrequently, depression is the result of medical treatment, for instance with hypotensive drugs such as methyldopa and reserpine, or excessive sedation. It is easy for the unwary to confuse depression with dementia, to assume that the disinterest of a depressed old lady is a sign of failing mental faculties. Even when there is evidence of early dementia, depression frequently coexists—understandably when the patient is still capable of recognising that her mental powers are beginning to decline—compounding the distress of patient and relatives. Endogenous depression, unipolar and bipolar types, can arise for the first time in old age, although with increasing rarity, but for the most part disorders of this nature are recurrences of earlier illness; age does not affect their frequency or severity.

Many minor states of anxiety and depression, frequently with a hypochondriacal colouring, are best treated with small doses of a neuroleptic, 1 mg trifluoperazine or 0·5 mg of haloperidol three times a day. Occasionally diazepam 2 to 5 mg is better, but very often the diazepine derivatives expose and exacerbate depression. However, they are satisfactory hypnotics at night; 15 mg flurazepam or 2·5 mg nitrazepam, for example.

When depression is more marked, and especially when the patient is agitated, and whether or not there are mild signs of dementia, an antidepressant is needed. Of the tricyclics we prefer dothiepin or doxepin, because their anticholinergic effects are relatively low. Given a 70-year-old patient, it is advisable to begin with 10 mg morning and night, and increase the dosage by 10 mg every other day to as near 150 mg a day as side effects will allow. Any sign of postural hypotension, or reports of confusion, are indications for lowering the dosage, at least for a time. The majority of depressed old people can reach 75 mg a day; best given two or even three times a day, to keep the concentration of the drug in the body as even as possible.

Provided depression is not severe, it is advisable to wait a month before assessing the full effect of the drug. If depression persists, because the drug is unsuitable, or the dosage inadequate because of side effects, it is best to change to another type of antidepressant; mianserin, which has the advantage of little anticholinergic activity, flupenthixol, tryptophan or, when depression is incapacitating, an MAOI such as tranylcypromine.

Tranylcypromine is most effective in patients who have always been anxious insecure people. It is as well to start with 10 mg a day, in the morning, and only increase to 10 mg twice a day after a week, provided there are no serious side effects. Improvement should be apparent after a fortnight's treatment. When results are disappointing, and particularly if early morning waking is a prominent symptom, it is worth combining a small dose of trimipramine, 10 to 25 mg at bedtime, with tranylcypromine. Great care is needed when treating old people with this combination, and it should be studiously avoided if there is any likelihood of confusion.

E.c.t. is a safe treatment, and can be given at any age. It should never be withheld if depression is at all severe, or in danger of becoming chronic. The contraindications are those listed on (p. 61). Osteoporosis is no hindrance, and merely calls for slightly more muscle relaxant than usual.

Lithium may be needed in old age, if manic depression then develops. The dosage is worked up slowly, starting with 250 mg a day, and increasing by this dose weekly until the serum concentration reaches 0·6 to 0·8 mmol/l. However, some old people are well controlled, and feel better, on a dosage which produces a serum concentration of 0·4 mmol/l or even lower. It is best to spread lithium over the day, rather than taking the drug in one dose at bedtime.

Cases of late schizophrenia are much less common. The majority present with well encapsulated paranoid symptoms, usually concerning neighbours. Neighbours are believed to watch or follow them, and sometimes bug their houses. In some instances, gases are pumped through the floor, rays directed on to them, and voices and noises are heard through the walls. First rank symptoms are frequenly absent, and there are no signs of dementia. Removal of the patient to hospital, or even to the peaceful home of a relative, is often enough to cause symptoms to fade and disappear, but a neuroleptic is equally effective; trifluoperazine 5 mg o.m., 10 mg o.n. (with an antiParkinsonian drug if necessary), lessens paranoid symptoms within a fortnight; after a month they are often gone. Inpatient treatment is only necessary if the patient is unco-operative over medication, or if much illfeeling and resentment towards the patient has been engendered in the neighbourhood. These patients tend to be isolated people, and not a few have some long-standing sensory impairment, often quite severe; deafness, or a visual defect. While it may be possible to improve these, it is not easy to persuade them to widen their lives. The neuroleptic drug has to be continued for at least a year, and often indefinitely, if paranoid symptoms are not to recur.

Depression often accompanies these paranoid states, and may lift as delusions fade. If depression is at all deep, or persists after delusional ideas have disappeared, treatment with antidepressant drugs, or even e.c.t., is necessary.

Dementia can begin at any age, but only becomes a serious medical problem from the sixties onwards. Very occasionally the underlying causes are treatable, vitamin B12 deficiency, hypothyroidism, a subdural haematoma, G.P.I., but for the most part the condition is progressive and uninfluenced by any treatment. There is certainly no good evidence that any of the so-called cerebral vasodilators can arrest intellectual decline. Nor, unless the patient has been living alone and neglecting himself, are injections of vitamin complexes needed.

The onset of dementia is insidious. Presenting symptoms vary widely between patients, depending on their basic personalities, the extent and site of the cortical disorder, and how much insight is retained; failing memory, irresponsible or antisocial behaviour, or depression severe enough for suicide to be attempted. It is inexcusable to overlook dementia, but equally inexcusable to ignore signs of depression and withhold treatment. Much can be done to improve the mood of a patient in the early stages, and give him, and especially his relatives, time to adjust to the inevitable. If depression is severe, e.c.t. may be called for, and given without fear of exacerbating the dementing process. It is of course essential for relatives to understand fully the situation, the reasons for treatment, and what to expect from it.

Periods of confusion are liable to develop at any stage, often precipitated by emotional strain, intercurrent infection, and not infrequently by drugs. If possible the latter should be stopped; reasonable clarity of mind should return within 24 hours. When the cause is infection, or family disruptions, haloperidol is probably the ideal drug to prescribe; 5 mg intramuscularly has a rapid calming effect, and is repeated after 6 hours, or if the patient is co-operative, followed by 1·5 mg orally every 4 to 6 hours. Chlorpromazine, and even thioridazine, are liable to increase or prolong confusion, as are the diazepine derivatives. As confusion clears, so the dosage of haloperidol is reduced and eventually stopped.

As dementia progresses the patient loses insight into his state, and becomes less and less able to cope with his everyday existence. His emotions become disinhibited. His mood is labile, and he weeps and becomes agitated easily. Antidepressant treatments are not helpful at this stage, and indeed are likely to do more harm than good. Neuroleptics help to reduce paranoid ideas, aggressive outbursts and agitation. Small doses of trifluoperazine 2 to 6 mg a day, or haloperidol 1 to 3 mg a day, are particularly useful in this respect. Thioridazine, the dose ranging from 25 to 100 mg, alone or with flurazepam 15 mg, ensures sleep and allows the patient's family to have undisturbed nights. If this is not effective, then it is worth trying chlormethiazole, 1 g with a hypnotic at bedtime.

Occasionally, when a patient is particularly difficult and tiresome at home, and cannot easily be controlled by drugs given orally, a small dose of a long-acting neuroleptic, 20 mg flupenthixol intramuscularly, or 10 mg fluphenazine, given monthly, is an effective tranquilliser, reducing agitation and improving mood and behaviour.

Too large a dose of any drug is liable to make the dementing patient confused, and add to his and his family's difficulties. Ideally the therapist should be in close touch with whoever is living with the patient, so that he hears quickly of any drug mishaps. As the patient declines, so his need for drugs lessens.

Most dementing old people are still cared for at home until the terminal stage, and their relatives need to be supported and advised. Day centres not only help to lessen and postpone deterioration in the patient's mood and behaviour, but also give his relatives a breathing space. Admitting the patient to hospital for a week or two, once or twice a year, also provides them with much needed relief.

FURTHER READING

Davies, G. 1978. Treatment in psychogeriatrics. In *Therapy Options in Psychiatry*. Ed. Connolly, J. Pitman Medical. England.

Kay, D.W.K. 1976. The depressions and neuroses of later life. In *Recent Advances in Clinical Psychiatry*. Ed. Granville-Grossman, K. Churchill Livingstone. Edinburgh.

11

Treatment of alcoholic and other addictions

ADDICTIONS OTHER THAN TO ALCOHOL

Although the number and varieties of addictions have been increasing in recent years, with more and more young people endangered, neither singly nor together do they create more than a small fraction of the social and medical problems caused by alcoholism.

The illegal use of cannabis, amphetamines, barbiturates, L.S.D., cocaine, heroin and other opiates has become fairly widespread. We may also reflect that the consumption of cigarettes has not diminished. Dependence on prescribed tranquillisers and sedatives is common, even if under medical control. Medical awareness of the danger of barbiturate dependence has greatly reduced prescriptions of these drugs, but it is still a serious problem.

Opiates

Addicts have to be handled with caution. If an unknown patient presents himself asking for a further supply of addictive drugs and claiming that he obtains them legally, it is wise to check with the doctor who prescribed for him previously, the dispensing chemist, or the Dangerous Drugs Branch of the Home Office. Blue-black needle tracks should be sought in those who claim to be mainliners. If possible the patient should be referred to a special drug dependency clinic for treatment and meanwhile only chlorpromazine in moderate dosage, and diphenoxylate hydrochloride prescribed. Drug addiction, by definition, is not in itself an emergency. However, particularly in hospital casualty departments, a patient may present with unequivocal signs of opiate withdrawal, i.e. anxiety, restlessness, sweating, a running nose and eyes, diarrhoea, vomiting and cramps, and the well known 'goose flesh', accompanied by weakness and craving for the drug. Blood pressure, pulse and respiration rates are all increased. In such cases methadone linctus 10 ml (4 mg) may be given hourly until symptoms subside. Only very rarely, because of severe vomiting, is it necessary to give methadone 10 mg intramuscularly.

Treatment of the drug user is never easy, for his motivation is all too often poor. He may seek treatment because of pressure from his family or at work, in the hope of escaping prosecution, or simply to obtain a further supply of the drug. Most addicts on opiates are treated in drug addiction centres. Although these units have been in existence for more than 12 years, their role and usefulness are still by no means clear. A number of patients on heroin do not want to come off their drugs totally. In such cases the policy is to switch from heroin to methadone. While withdrawal symptoms from heroin occur within 12 hours, methadone 'lasts' for 24 hours, enabling a night's sleep. It produces less euphoria and is therefore rather less addictive than heroin. Nonetheless, many patients become dependent on their regular daily dosage of methadone. One mg methadone is equivalent to 1 mg heroin, 3 mg morphine, 20 mg pethidine, and 30 mg codeine. Unlike heroin, no Home Office licence is needed to prescribe methadone to addicts.

For optimum success in withdrawing a patient from opiates he must be in hospital, isolated from his addicted friends. Methadone replaces heroin, and is then reduced at the rate of 10 mg less each 48 hours. Tranquillisers such as chlorpromazine and chlormethiazole are usually given at first, and tricyclic antidepressants may be useful later. If withdrawal on an outpatient basis is attempted, each 10 mg step requires at least 2 weeks. The patient's morale has to be built up, and he must be helped to organise his life in a more realistic and ultimately satisfying way. Individual psychotherapy, based on a strong transference between therapist and patient is most important, as is group psychotherapy. Follow-up treatment must be continued for a minimum of a year and usually considerably longer. Rehabilitation is a long drawn-out process, and during the early part of it the patient may need a specialised hostel in which to live. Relapse is common, but should not cause the therapist to give up, provided the patient still shows motivation.

Barbiturates and stimulants

The extent of addiction and habituation to barbiturates is hard to assess. Most neurotic patients, who previously needed barbiturate sedation for their symptoms, now receive a diazepine derivative. But from time to time one sees patients who are taking very large doses regularly, obtaining these supplies from several doctors, each unaware of the other's prescriptions. The treatment of an addiction of this kind is usually fairly easy, unless the patient has a very abnormal personality, or large amounts have been taken for too long. Withdrawal must always be gradual, otherwise there is a risk of increasing anxiety, cardiovascular collapse, epileptic fits, and confusion; a state similar to delirium tremens, and equally dangerous.

Amphetamine is often taken by barbiturate and alcoholic addicts to wake themselves up. Others who come to use increasing doses of amphetamines include adolescents, for weekend jags, and neurotic women who began by asking for slimming tablets. There is little doubt that the combination of amphetamine and amylo-barbitone is particularly liable to cause addiction. Toxic psychoses, resembling schizophrenia, may occur when more than 50 mg daily of amphetamine is habitually consumed. A urine test is useful in confirming the diagnosis.

All stimulant drugs, including methylphenidate and cocaine, can be stopped immediately, since no physical withdrawal symptoms occur, although depression and irritability are often troublesome for some days and require sedation. Sometimes an antidepressant is also helpful, and it will prevent the craving from becoming overpowering in the months following withdrawal of the drug.

Hallucinogens

L.S.D. may produce a psychotic state with hallucinations, acute anxiety, severe panic, depression or a toxic confusional state. Such symptoms are best treated in a hospital ward with intramuscular chlorpromazine or haloperidol. 'Flashback' symptoms, resembling those of a bad trip, may recur for a year or so after stopping L.S.D.; in particular, panics and visual distortions are common. Diazepam, or even chlorpromazine, may be required; and above all, reassurance.

Marihuana smoking is now common. Usually there is a period of stimulation followed by sedation lasting about 6 hours; but there is wide individual variation in the response to the drug. Effects are unpredictable, and range from elation to panic or depression. There is usually vasodilatation of the face capillaries; pupillary dilatation, and a rise in heart rate and blood pressure. Perceptual changes, including synaesthesiae, illusions and hallucinations, may occur and experience of time altered. Severe adverse reactions may require immediate treatment with chlorpromazine or haloperidol, but the majority can be dealt with by 10 to 20 mg of diazepam orally, repeated after 2 hours if necessary. The tranquillisers may need to be continued for some weeks while underlying emotional problems are dealt with. While some of those who use cannabis *excessively* have disordered personalities, the majority are immature young people.

DEPENDENCE ON ALCOHOL

The evils of addiction to alcohol are of a higher order of magnitude than those caused by the drugs we have mentioned, both in social extent and threat to mental and physical health. The fact that the only limitation on the consumption of alcohol is the depth of the consumer's pocket has meant that in all countries and at all times alcoholism has remained a major social and medical problem. It is out of the virtues of alcohol that its dangers arise. Taken in reasonable amounts and at suitable times, its influence is largely beneficial; its disinhibiting effects are valuable in social converse and in taking the edge off many of life's unavoidable tensions. The fact that, though helpful to the many it may be disastrous to a substantial minority, has often prompted the demand that its use be prohibited or strictly controlled. When this has been tried, however, the disadvantages have proved more far-reaching than the advantages.

A large number of people enjoy alcohol and come to no harm. No discussion of the treatment of alcoholism is worth while until the group who may be seriously endangered is more clearly defined. Many people who drink alcohol go through life without running into excess. Those who do can be classified into three groups, which to a certain extent overlap. The occasional and reasonable drinker may now and again overstep the mark. Usually no harm is done, but sometimes it happens that in a drunken state he offends against the law, perhaps with very serious personal consequences. For a time in this country there were large numbers of men who got drunk reguarly once a week on pay-day. Today, the working man spends more time at home, perhaps watching television, while alcohol excess is likelier in the young 'expense account' drinker. The problem here is mainly a social and legal one; medical complications are not common in this group.

Secondly, there is the heavy and steady drinker, who may become dependent on the drug but does not lose his ability to keep its consumption under control. The addiction, in fact, is not compulsive. He is quite able to reduce the amount he takes if he is convinced that it is necessary, though he may be a little hard to persuade. The amount he takes may be a financial drain, and in course of time his physical and mental health may begin to suffer; but he does not appear drunk on important occasions, or pull down his life in ruins in the course of a few months. While the capacity for control is still present, and the addiction is reversible, treatment once begun in a co-operative spirit is fairly easy. The main danger arises from the fact that if consumption has been heavy over a long time, changes may have taken place in the nervous system and in the personality, which may prove irreversible. As well, and earlier in women than men, progressive liver damage may develop. A certain proportion of drinkers in this class graduate into the third group.

It is the third group which provides the main problem, for in their case treatment is urgently needed, is often exceptionally difficult, yet may be outstandingly successful. The drinkers in this class are those who, once started, seem unable to stop drinking until drunkenness supervenes. The predisposition to this reaction may be acquired, for instance, after a head injury, or even after damage to the constitution from a more normal type of over-indulgence in alcohol. But very often it seems to have a genetic basis. Twin and adoption studies give some support to this. Positive family histories are often obtained if carefully inquired for. A son may be a teetotaller, having seen his father or mother develop the disease, but fails then to confide the true reason to his own children, who in turn fall prey to the condition. The chances of anyone with an alcoholic parent becoming an alcoholic is about one in four. Social and environmental factors also play a part. A society like ours which encourages drinking as an aid to social intercourse and relaxation brings to light a high proportion of its members constitutionally at risk.

Compulsive drinking may start early or late in life. The man affected is often noted in his youth for a particularly hard head; he can out-drink his friends without showing undue effects—though even early on he may show a tendency, after a certain amount of alcohol has been taken, to continue drinking when the normal drinker will stop. Later, and this may vary from a few months to several years, loss of control occurs, which is the hallmark of addiction. From here the alcoholic travels steadily and inevitably down the road to disaster. Now the first drink taken sets up a pathological and irresistible craving for more, which continues until supplies run out or the drinker becomes inebriated. With increasing age and impaired hepatic efficiency, diminishing tolerance develops and ever smaller quantities of alcohol cause intoxication. At first the alcoholic is still able to decide whether or not he begins to drink at any one time. Characteristically, these patients can recall how they went 'on the water wagon' for long spells after a particularly heavy or prolonged drinking bout, or drinking disaster. But as time goes by these 'dry periods' become ever shorter and finally cease. Withdrawal effects become increasingly frequent and severe, until alcohol is required immediately on waking, and at intervals throughout the day.

Social and economic factors now intrude as the alcoholic tries to arrange his life around his drinking. He drinks secretly, drops his friends, becomes increasingly disinhibited, quarrels with his family, perhaps loses his job. His libido diminishes and he may begin to behave jealously towards his wife. 'Blackouts' and other forms of memory disturbance become prominent. Even a few drinks so impair memory retention that next day he is unable to remember anything of the previous night. Capacity for recent recall, judgment and insight are affected even when sober. A marked change of personality develops. Insomnia, hallucinations, and increasing waves of fear may herald the approach of delirium tremens and impending disaster. Finally a stage may be reached when the taking of quite small quantities of alcohol leads to the abrogation of all judgment and control, and a catastrophe is inevitable.

When a patient of this kind comes for treatment it must be made absolutely clear both to him and his relatives that there is no immediate alternative to complete abstinence, however it is obtained. The failure of treatment will be ensured if the doctor tries to put the compulsive drinker on a ration of alcohol. Such half measures may be tried only with the controlled but steady drinker who has been overdoing it.

The compulsive drinker always needs some psychological preparation before beginning treatment. He must be convinced that total and *permanent* abstinence is his only hope for the future, and that a cure of his idiosyncrasy, permitting him to 'drink normally', or even to have an occasional drink, is impossible. It is justifiable, but generally futile, to appeal to his moral sense, and his sense of responsibility toward his family. It is more effective to stress the very real dangers of physical disease, dementia, social degradation and death, that may result from alcohol. Until the alcoholic realises his plight and is prepared to co-operate fully in the treatment, it is generally useless to undertake it. It is better to tell the patient to go away and return when his inevitable downward progress has at last convinced him that nothing but treatment followed by total abstinence will save him from the gutter. Agreement to a 6 month period without alcohol, and then to review the situation, is a minimum requirement for starting treatment.

All physical and psychological treatments of compulsive alcoholism have this single aim, of bringing about a stable habit of abstinence. The selection of one method rather than another depends on the special skills of the therapist, and on the personality, circumstances, and particular needs of the patient.

Treatment

Although the well motivated and physically fit alcoholic can be satisfactorily treated as an outpatient, most patients with established alcohol dependence need to start their treatment in hospital. Not only is it difficult to control severe withdrawal symptoms and to prevent delirium tremens, but the heavy drinker cannot be relied on to stop drinking unless removed from his familiar drinking surroundings and temptations. Even if he still has a devoted family, it is not fair to expect them to endure the strain and responsibility of supervising him. Once he has agreed to treatment, no time should be lost in admitting him. The common early withdrawal symptoms are tremor, sweating, nausea, sleep disturbance, often associated with vivid dreams, and depression of mood. If delirium tremens develops over the first 3 or 4 days, perception becomes increasingly disturbed, culminating in terrifying visual and sometimes auditory hallucinations and confusion, especially at night.

There are many ways of 'drying out' a patient. We favour one of the diazepines, and prefer lorazepam because of its quick action, uncomplicated metabolism, and relatively short half-life. This allows a change of dosage to have a rapid effect. If the patient is tremulous or distressed an intravenous injection of 4 mg is given initially to settle him. After that 2·5 mg is given every 4 hours, but may be increased to 5 mg if necessary. Withdrawal symptoms are well controlled on this dosage and the patient is drowsy; he is kept in bed. This regime is continued for 5 days. The dose of lorazepam is then reduced progressively. The patient is allowed up on 1 mg three times a day. He may require a hypnotic at night for a while.

The diazepines have the advantage of not depressing respiration or causing stupor, and of being unlikely to produce dependence in the short term. There is probably little difference between the efficacy of the different derivatives, but it is as well for the therapist to familiarise himself with a particular one. If a patient is disorientated, disturbed and uncooperative, or is vomiting because of gastritis, the drug must be given parenterally; 4 mg lorazepam or 15 mg diazepam, given intravenously if possible, has a rapid tranquillising effect.

A number of other drugs have their advocates and disadvantages. The neuroleptics have long been used. Haloperidol, 20 to 40 mg parenterally, is useful for quickly gaining control of an obstreperous patient (see p. 40), but is unsatisfactory for providing continuous control. Chlorpromazine is better in this respect, but has the disadvantage of increasing the likelihood of fits. Other phenothiazines, such as promazine or thioridazine, are not as effective.

Chlormethiazole is without doubt effective in controlling alcoholic withdrawal symptoms, but it carries the risk of dependence if continued for more than a week or so after the patient has been withdrawn. Barbital, a long-acting barbiturate, excreted unchanged through the kidney, is still recommended by some authorities. However, we endorse the majority view that barbiturates are best avoided, in view of their tendency to depress respiration and consciousness, and their dependence potential, and, occasionally, they cause paradoxical excitement.

Other drugs still used include paraldehyde, an excellent drug were it not for its smell, and the liability to abscess formation when given intramuscularly. Alcohol itself controls most withdrawal symptoms, but not delirium tremens once this has developed. Some authorities still give diminishing amounts for the first 3 or 4 days of withdrawal treatment.

As important as the tranquillising effect of drugs is the general management and care of the patient. The mortality rate was once high, and is still not insignificant, largely because insufficient care was devoted to the patient's physical state. Many patients are in poor condition on admission, and need to be carefully renourished. It is sensible, and sometimes essential, to give vitamins parenterally, especially those of the B complex. Intestinal absorption of thiamine may be impaired, even when a full diet is taken. The usual procedure is to give a daily injection of B and C vitamins in high dosage for the first 5 days (large doses of thiamine remove any risk of Wernicke's encephalopathy). Phenytoin is sometimes advocated in the hope of preventing fits, but we feel this to be unnecessary when a benzodiazepine is employed. Physical disease must be looked for, and treated if present. The patient needs to be quiet and sleepy, but it is important for him to keep in touch with his surroundings as much as possible; he must understand what is happening to him and why, and feel that he is in friendly surroundings.

Withdrawal symptoms improve after a few days, but may not disappear completely for a fortnight. When they have been severe, and particularly if delirium tremens has supervened, mental functioning does not completely return to normal for about a month; capacity for insight and conceptual thought are slow to return, and too much must not be expected from psychotherapy during this early period. In some cases of delirium tremens the patient may be left with permanent brain damage.

Treatment of established alcoholism

Subsequent management must be tailored to the patient's motivation and personality, his life style, problems and circumstances. There is no one treatment for alcoholism. It is essential to learn as much about the patient as possible before deciding on a therapeutic plan. Close relatives or friends may be able to provide important information, and should be seen whenever practical. Their understanding of and co-operation in the patient's treatment may be a vital factor for its success.

As we have already said, lasting benefit is unlikely to result for the majority of alcoholics unless they are prepared to give up alcohol completely. Some patients cannot accept the idea of never drinking again, and with them it may be reasonable to strike a bargain; 6 months' abstinence followed by a trial period of controlled drinking. Much depends on the patient's resolution and character. When these are strong the patient may indeed be able to adjust his attitude and drinking habits in such a way as to allow him to drink comparatively normally. Even so, relapses are likely under periods of strain, and it is important that the patient trusts his doctor sufficiently to seek guidance immediately in such an event and not allow alcoholism to re-establish itself.

Much can be done to help the controlled drinker by commonsense advice and encouragement, and the setting of limits. For instance, perhaps he should not drink outside certain hours, or only at mealtimes; never on his own, or at weekends only; or never at business engagements, and so on. Failure to follow the agreed rules must be carefully noted by the patient, the reasons discussed and recognised and a lesson learned. The more the patient willingly accepts responsibility for his behaviour, and recognises the danger signs, the more hopeful the outlook.

Biofeedback techniques (see p. 94) help some patients; they monitor the level of alcohol in their blood, by the use of a breathalyser, and learn to restrict their intake so that blood alcohol levels never rise above, say, 60 mg per cent.

Aversion therapy was widely used in the past, and still has a place today (see p. 89). Patients need to be carefully selected and, needless to say, must all be strongly motivated to give up alcohol totally and indefinitely. They are mostly over 35, and compulsive drinkers, of a good, usually driving, obsessional personality, with stable, successful work records, and with satisfactory social lives before these began to be affected by their drinking. Aversion therapy is not generally successful with younger patients, whose drinking is likely to reflect their inadequacy and unsatisfactory lives. Other methods are better for them.

Aversion therapy utilises classical conditioning, linking obnoxious experience with the consumption of alcohol. Unpleasant electric shocks are given through electrodes attached to the patient's forearm, immediately he begins to drink, or imagines himself doing so. About 20 aversion pairing trials are carried out at each daily session, and the treatment lasts for a week. In fact, electric shock methods give disappointing results in alcoholism, and are nothing like as effective as emetic drug-induced aversion. The effect of nausea and vomiting after drinking has a more powerful aversive effect than electric shocks, perhaps because the mouth plays so large a part in the alcoholic's drinking rituals. In addition to deconditioning the patient, emetic aversion therapy produces a state of physical debility and heightened suggestibility, allowing old patterns of thought to be broken up and new ones substituted. It seems that until comparatively recently, behaviour therapists failed to take the cognitive aspects of treatment into consideration. How the patient views his treatment and his experiences during it, is just as important as the formation of a conditioned aversion to alcohol.

A psychological build up to aversion treatment is a necessary preliminary. If the patient is to be helped to make a fundamental change in his way of life, every relevant factor in his personality and situation must be utilised. During the 5 or 6 days of treatment he must be isolated from all his former drinking associations, however tenuous; it is advisable therefore to forbid all visitors and telephone calls.

One particular doctor should conduct treatment throughout. He must know as much as possible about the patient's background, and particularly the kind of situation which tempts him to drink. Incidents in his past life, connected with his drinking, about which he feels particularly ashamed, should be explored in detail. These will be used again later, during the actual aversion treatment. A test dose of 0·3 mg apomorphine is given intramuscularly the day before, to check for particular sensitivity.

Suggestibility can be heightened by keeping the room in semi-darkness and spotlighting bottles of alcohol placed at the foot of the bed. Three mg apomorphine is injected intramuscularly. The patient sits in bed with a blanket over his shoulders and a vomiting bowl at hand. The pulse rate should be recorded every 3 minutes, and the blood pressure at 5 minute intervals, until vomiting begins. Five minutes after the injection, when the patient is beginning to feel queasy, the first drink is poured out with due formality and handed to the patient. The glass is warmed by placing it in hot water, so that the smell of the drink is enhanced. A suitable drink is 30 ml whisky or gin, or the equivalent of whatever the patient's preferred drink is, diluted with half as much warm water. He is told to smell it for a full 2 minutes and remember the pleasures of the past, the pleasure of the first drink of the day, the relief of tension, the escape from the sense of responsibility; all the information the therapist has gained about the patient can now be used. He must then take a mouthful, hold it for a minute or two, and then swallow it slowly. He will rapidly vomit.

Under such psychological pressure the patient may at first defend himself, even pugnaciously, but once vomiting starts, what is left of his morale collapses. At this point, when he is feeling his most miserable and suggestibility is at a maximum, the therapist must offer him support and hope of recovery. He is told that he has the ability to recreate his life and to restore his self-respect, but only if he shuns the first drink. He must be aware that he will always be one drink away from ruin; he can never drink in the future. In this respect he is different from other men, and no compromise is possible. Either he gives up drink for ever and lives again, or his first drink is his last as a free man, and he sinks into the gutter.

It is important to give the first drink before nausea begins, for otherwise the conditioned aversion to alcohol will be weakened. If vomiting does not occur within 5 minutes of taking the first drink, a further 3 mg apomorphine should be given intramuscularly. This will quickly produce results. Usually four or five drinks are given quickly, sometimes ending with 230 ml of warm ale, containing 60 mg of ipecacuanha, to prolong nausea.

Nausea may persist for an hour or more after vomiting has ceased. The patient is left alone in bed for 2 hours, the bottles of alcohol placed in front of him. After this, if blood pressure and pulse are satisfactory, he gets up and is allowed to mix with other patinets.

Six treatments on successive days are given, but it is advisable to have a day of rest in the middle. Complications are rare. Marked and persistent hypotension and tachycardia are indications that treatment should be stopped.

Disulfiram has been used since 1949 in the treatment of alcoholism. The drug interferes with the breakdown of alcohol, causing acetaldehyde to accumulate in the body, with unpleasant consequences. Occasionally these are severe, and even fatal, and it is therefore important to select patients carefully before prescribing the drug. Needless to say disulfiram does not cure, nor does it remove the desire for alcohol—it works entirely through fear.

Disulfiram has a long action, and one dose a day, 200 to 400 mg, taken in the morning, is enough to provide cover for 24 to 72 hours. If the alcoholic drinks during this period he develops some of the following symptoms within 10 to 15 minutes; flushing, tachycardia and palpitations, constriction of the chest, pounding headache, nausea and sometimes vomiting, and intense fear of impending death. Hypotension may be marked, and occasionally leads to cardiovascular collapse and myocardial infarction. Hangover effects may last for many hours. The more alcohol consumed the greater these effects are likely to be.

The drug is not therefore suitable for alcoholics whose ability to control their sudden impulses is poor and who cannot be relied upon not to drink through the disulfiram. It is the strongly motivated patient, often somewhat obsessional, who feels protected once he has taken his daily tablet of disulfiram, who benefits, knowing that if he drinks the consequences are likely to be devastating.

It is as well to give most patients a disulfiram challenge at the start of treatment. Needless to say, a history of heart disease and cirrhosis are absolute contraindications. An e.c.g. is advisable before beginning treatment. The patient, who can be an outpatient, receives 600 mg of disulfiram a day for 2 days, 400 mg a day over the next 2 days, and on the day of the challenge 200 mg. He is then given 30 ml whisky, or half a pint of beer, repeated every 15 minutes if there is no immediate effect, up to 120 ml whisky. The reaction is occasionally delayed up to 2 hours after the first drink.

If the reaction is unduly severe 1 g ascorbic acid (involved in the oxidation of acetaldehyde), and phenergan 50 mg are given intravenously (since part of the reaction is due to the release of histamine).

Side effects of disulfiram are sometimes troublesome; acneform eruptions, halitosis, gastro-intestinal disturbances, fatigue, headache, peripheral neuropathy, reduced sexual potency and, rarely, psychotic episodes and depression. Symptoms due to the absence of alcohol may be blamed onto the drug by the patient.

Citrated calcium carbide has similar but milder effects to disulfiram. Its length of action is shorter, 12 hours, and the drug must be taken twice a day; the dose is 50 to 100 mg.

The disadvantage of both these drugs is that their efficacy depends on the patient taking the drug each day. If he wakes up and decides to drink on that or the next day, he merely omits the drug. A few patients learn to drink their way through the drug's effects, and clearly derive a sense of triumph from this achievement. There is no point in continuing disulfiram in such an event.

However, the majority of patients on disulfiram, or citrated calcium carbide, have a healthy respect for its interaction with alcohol, and only drink when off the drug for at least 1 day. To overcome the difficulty of drug compliance, subcutaneous implants of disulfiram have been given, which are claimed to last for about 6 months. In fact the effect of these implants is more psychological than pharmacological for the release of disulfiram into the blood stream is erratic, and often too low to interfere effectively with the metabolism of alcohol. The ideal patient for implantation is one who is terrified of drinking while on disulfiram; he dare not risk drinking, and feels secure for 6 months. In suitable cases another implant can be inserted at the end of this time.

Tranquillisers and antidepressants are often necessary at some stage of a patient's treatment. Particularly when treating the young, tense, insecure alcoholic, a tranquilliser may be needed in place of alcohol if he is to cope with his responsibilities and continue to lead his normal life. Diazepam, or one of its analogues, is the most satisfactory drug for this purpose, but care must be taken that it is not abused.

Depression is commonly experienced by alcoholics, particularly those of middle age. Depression reduces their motivation and increases the likelihood of their drinking. An antidepressant drug is indicated in such cases. The dose need not be large. Sleep is often disturbed when alcohol is stopped, and amitriptyline or trimipramine at bedtime can counteract this, as well as depression. In those patients who have used alcohol for many years in order to overcome a chronic state of tension and reactive depression, a combination of Parstelin in the day and trimipramine at night is often most effective. How long these drugs need to be given depends on the patient's ability to adapt to a life without alcohol.

It is claimed that a few periodic drinkers are helped by lithium. When excessive drinking stems from recurring affective disorders, it is certainly reasonable to prescribe lithium. But in fact few periodic drinkers show clear evidence of this. Depressive symptoms are often secondary to heavy drinking, and disappear once alcohol is abandoned; or, more frequently, they are a reflection of chronic tension. It seems probably that many of the apparent successes with lithium occur in younger patients with aggressive personality disorders. Lithium may exert a nonspecific dulling effect on such patients.

The success of physical treatments of alcoholism depends on adequate follow-up and the application of all available methods to maintain teetotalism or controlled drinking. Psychotherapy begins from the first meeting with the patient, provided withdrawal symptoms are not severe, when the therapist explores the reasons for the patient's drinking, and discusses how he may avoid temptation in the future. The trust and confidence the patient has in his therapist is of immense importance; a major drawback at many alcoholic clinics is the system by which patients are seen by different doctors at different stages in their progress, ultimately leading to a feeling that there is no therapeutic continuity.

Frequently the patient has problems in his home life, perhaps the result of his drinking, with which he must be helped. Close relatives must be seen, singly or with the patient, depending on circumstances. In any case, it is vital to assess the stability of the patient's family from the start, for it is often on the brink of disintegration by the time he comes for treatment.

Group therapy is helpful to many but not all alcoholics in understanding themselves and their need to drink, and in providing mutual support and protection. Meetings once or twice a week, preferably after work, may usefully continue for a year or more. Groups may be run on the principle of the 'confessional', patients describing their past misdeeds, or along more conventional psychotherapeutic lines, including the inculcation of social skills. Many patients benefit from joining Alcoholics Anonymous, a voluntary organisation run by alcoholics for alcoholics. There are branches all over Great Britain and in the United States. Here patients meet others who will accept and encourage them.

AL-ANON exists for the relatives and close friends of alcoholics, organises meetings, and provides considerable support for families who, in the past, felt helpless and lost.

Other voluntary bodies who cater for the needs of alcoholics are the Church Army, the Church of England Temperance Society, the Reginald Carter Foundation, the Joseph Rowntree Social Service Trust, the Helping Hand and the Salvation Army.

Treatment of the chronic drunken offender

Each day, on an average, the courts in the United Kingdom deal with some 200 drunken offences. In the past these drunks, usually homeless, jobless and friendless, revolved through court, prison, drunkenness, court, ad infinitum, a degrading, expensive, recurring, futile procedure. Now rehabilitation, instead of repeated prison sentences, is being attempted by means of detoxication centres, and 'skid row' hostels. Whether this form of treatment proves successful will depend on the amount of support the community is prepared to extend to these patients, the quality of therapy provided, and the degree of motivation it is possible to induce.

FURTHER READING

Clare, A.W., 1979. The causes of alcoholism. *Brit. J. Hosp. Med.* April. 403.

Hemmingsen, R., Kramp, P., Rafaelsen, O.J. 1979. Delirium tremens. *Acta Psychiatrica Scandinavica*. **59**. 337.

Leader. 1977. How important are genetic influences on alcohol dependence? *Brit. Med. J.* **2**. 1371.

12

Child psychiatry

A child, compared to an adult, is more malleable, more strongly influenced by family and social forces. This stems from his dependency, at first total on others, and because his central nervous system continues to develop and remain receptive and modifiable.

A child's development dates from conception. He inherits certain characteristics and potentials in respect of temperament and intelligence. How these shape and finally form depend on a continuous dynamic interplay between his environment and his genetic endowment.

He comes under many influences. Increasingly a child influences his world and provides a feedback to those concerned with him. An irritable, difficult child, or one who fails to respond normally to those around him, creates tension and dissatisfaction, particularly in his mother at first, and vice versa.

The infant has relatively few needs at first. Many of our present day concepts of child development stem from the work of Freud and his followers. Valuable as this has been, psychoanalytical attitudes have sometimes tended to hinder progress in child psychiatry. Mothers have been cast in the role of universal villain. The significance of a child's symptoms and behaviour, from a long-term point of view, has been ignored or looked at from a purely theoretical angle, and the form and value of treatment has been accepted dogmatically and uncritically. Only comparatively recently have we begun to collect information about how common some symptoms are at different stages of development, and their significance and relationship, if any, to later psychiatric disturbances. Prospective studies of patients who have attended psychiatric clinics have been and are being done. Epidemiology has provided information about the frequency of symptoms among the child population at various ages. Useful data has come from twin studies and surveys of children brought up in orphanages and foster homes. In the past decade ethology has provided a stimulus, although such concepts as 'critical learning periods' still lack evidence applicable to human development, and often ignore the important role of culture in the development of the human.

A major problem in child psychiatry concerns diagnosis. Only recently have child psychiatrists begun to agree about the need for classification of childhood disorders. Classification does not necessarily imply the existence of disease entities. A child is continually developing and classification must take this into account. Similar problems may manifest themselves in different ways at different ages. Rutter has emphasised the need for a classification based on fact rather than theoretical concepts, with predictive values.

Examination of the child and parents

Anxious parents bring their child to a doctor for reasons which often seem on the surface to be trivial. The practitioner must be able to recognise whether a child's behaviour is within normal limits. He must also have the wit to appreciate that parents may really be seeking help for their own problems rather than their child's.

One of the more obvious differences between child and adult psychiatry is that it is not the child but his parents who seek advice. In a sense therefore, parents are dissatisfied with their child and ready to hand him over to an expert. Many parents are liable to feel guilty and anxious. They may try to compensate for this by strong protective feelings for their child and criticism of the doctor.

A child's symptoms and behaviour frequently reflect family problems. Therefore, in addition to a history of the child's symptoms, adequate information about the personal and socio-economic history of the family must be obtained. A comprehensive interview may have a profound therapeutic effect on the parents, releasing tensions and inhibitions, and allowing them to see their child in a new light.

The examination of a child depends to some extent on his age. It is nearly always possible to get a reasonable history from children of 3 or 4 upwards, provided the questions are framed in a way which the child can understand. Initially it may be advisable to discuss some neutral topic, a game or television programme, and then gradually shift towards the child's problems. If this results in signs of anxiety the conversation can temporarily turn back to neutral ground. A good deal of information may be gained from observing a child's reactions to what is said. For the young inhibited child it may be helpful to ask him to draw a house, a human figure, or a wild animal. Not only may this picture relate to the child's difficulties but it can also serve as a talking point. Alternatively, he can be shown a picture and asked to comment on it. It is not usually necessary to use toys, but occasionally plasticine, sand, toy soldiers and so on are useful for drawing out a withdrawn child.

Adolescents, once their shyness or resentment is lost, are for the most part able to give a good account of themselves and their families, and to relate warmly to the therapist, unless psychotic or autistic, and it is not difficult to make a diagnosis and recognise the psychodynamics.

The vast majority of disturbed children are either suffering from neurotic inhibitory states, anxieties, phobias, depression, hypochondriasis, obsessions and tics, or 'acting out' disorders which arouse social disapproval. Psychotic illness and childhood autism are comparatively rare.

With neurotic and 'acting out' disorders, treatment for the most part aims to break a vicious circle; to help parents become aware of their child's individuality and needs, and enable the child to find a way out of the maze of resentment, guilt and depression in which he is trapped, and regain his self-confidence. Therapists vary in their approach. Some rely solely on psychotherapy; techniques range from frequent sessions with the child on his own, to family therapy, when everyone is included. Alternatively the psychotherapist may concentrate on one or other parent. Behaviour therapy and retraining methods have a useful part to play; particularly in treating enuresis and encopresis, and in phobic states, especially school phobia. Occasionally, when the home atmosphere is dreadful or the child's behaviour impossibly destructive, drastic measures such as residential care may have to be considered.

Treatment with drugs is not given as often as in adult psychiatry. Nonetheless, drugs are often able to banish a child's symptoms quickly, provide him with a good night's sleep, and restore tranquillity to a family increasingly disrupted by the child's behaviour. Yet not a few child psychiatrists still eschew drugs on the grounds that these deal only with the child's symptoms, not their causes. Of course the therapist must try to modify or remove the cause of the trouble, but that is no reason for not interrupting a child's symptoms as soon as possible, allowing him perhaps to get back to school, and bringing quick relief to the family; a drug, used wisely and for a short time, can sometimes achieve far more than a year of psychotherapy. But it is anachronistic to consider different methods of treatment as mutually exclusive; they are interchangeable and additive in their effects.

Anxiolytics like the diazepine derivatives are most effective in relieving anxiety in older children and adolescents. They are liable to cause children under the age of 8 or 9 to become drowsy in the daytime, and thereby interfere with school work and outside activities. However, they are sometimes able to relieve those abdominal pains, headaches, and sore throats, which occur repeatedly in some children from about 5 years onwards in response to emotional conflict, and for which no organic cause can be found. A diazepine is a valuable aid in the treatment of school phobia, and enables the 11-year-old boy to go to school on his own, so preventing the complications which develop if he is away from school for long, or if his mother always has to accompany him there. A single dose at bedtime, 5 mg, may be all that is required, the drug's tranquillising effect lasting throughout the next morning.

Diazepines are often given for sleeplessness. Again, they are most useful in older children and adolescents. Young children often refuse to go to sleep because they are anxious, develop elaborate rituals at bedtime, and insist that mother be present in the room. Such behaviour is often strengthened by the parents' responses; excessive anger, staying with the child for hours, or allowing him to come into the parental bed. A diazepine's action is not rapid enough in these cases, and the child is all too often able to resist its effects; the end result is a fractious child and an exhausted, exasperated parent. Chloral hydrate is still the most effective drug for producing sleep rapidly at any age, and its short action avoids hangover effects; 500 mg will send a 4-year-old soundly to sleep within 10 to 15 minutes.

Small doses of a phenothiazine derivative are able to relieve anxiety at all ages, and are particularly indicated when associated with anorexia. Ten mg chlorpromazine as syrup, three times a day before meals, calms a tense, resentful child, and encourages him to eat. In the young adolescent female this picture may develop into anorexia nervosa, when larger doses of chlorpromazine may be required (see p. 119). Ten to 25 mg chlorpromazine gives an anxious 10-year-old a good night's sleep. But promazine 25 mg is a better drug for insomnia at all ages, and is less likely to cause hangover effects.

Other neuroleptics, notably haloperidol, are sometimes effective in the treatment of tics, and particularly in that unusual condition, the Gilles de la Tourette syndrome; the dosage varies from 1·5 to 10 mg a day, depending on age.

Neuroleptics are also prescribed to hyperkinetic children. The hyperkinetic syndrome is probably made up from a number of conditions with different causes, and no one treatment is likely to be universally effective. Some children improve remarkably well with amphetamine or methylphenidate; overactivity is reduced and the child's attention span increased.

Barbiturates are not to be recommended for childhood psychiatric disorders. Children can tolerate large doses of barbiturates, and they may, paradoxically, cause restlessness and 'acting out' behaviour to increase.

Tricyclic antidepressants are valuable in the treatment of primary nocturnal enuresis, and they also have striking sedative and tranquillising effects on children. In fact these drugs are sometimes more satisfactory in this respect than the tranquillisers themselves. The dosage must be kept low, not more than 30 mg for a 10-year-old, the larger dose at bedtime. It may well be that depression lurks behind the anxiety of these children, as Eva Frommer maintained in the last edition of this book. We ourselves take the view that while depression of mood is extremely common in childhood and adolescence, this is very different from adult types of depressive illness; it is mostly always in response to environmental difficultires, and lifts quickly once these can be surmounted.

Manic depressive psychosis is rare, and indeed many authorities claim that it does not occur in childhood. Mania is certainly exceptional, and case reports of its occurrence do not clearly distinguish the condition from hyperkinetic states and childhood schizophrenia.

However, manic depression occurs with steadily increasing frequency once puberty is reached. Depression or mania may be the first manifestation; the latter is easily confused with, and mistaken for, a behaviour disorder. An important diagnostic pointer is a strong family history of bipolar affective illness.

Depression responds well to an antidepressant drug, and it is rare for a young adolescent to need e.c.t. Mania, when severe, requires treatment with haloperidol or chlorpromazine. Large doses usually need the addition of an antiParkinsonian drug.

Lithium is effective at any age, and should not be withheld from an adolescent or a child after a second attack of depression or mania. The stability of mood produced by the drug allows the patient to develop emotionally and academically during a vitally important period. The dosage must be adjusted carefully to suit the individual rather than according to arbitary serum lithium levels. It is as well to continue lithium until examinations are finished before attempting to stop the drug.

Childhood schizophrenia is uncommon, occurs mainly after the age of 8 or 9, and is often difficult to distinguish from progressive neurological disease. The aetiology is obscure, and there is no convincing evidence that child and adult schizophrenia are related. Treatment with a neuroleptic, a phenothiazine or thioxanthene derivative, or haloperidol, helps in a limited way only. These drugs merely control disturbed behaviour; they will not cure the child. The prognosis is extremely gloomy.

Childhood autism is unrelated to schizophrenia. First described by Kanner in 1943, the syndrome has been extended by Wing to include children whose initial development was apparently normal, the first signs not appearing until the second or third year of life. Drugs have little place in the treatment of this condition. However, tranquillisers are useful from time to time; whether a diazepine or neuroleptic derivative depends on individual reactions to each drug. Anticonvulsants may also be needed to control fits. Behaviour modification, aimed particularly at speech development and socialisation of the autistic child is sometimes helpful; much depends on the co-operation of the child's family and his teachers.

FURTHER READING

Graham, P. 1976. Management in child psychiatry. *Brit. J. Psychiat.* **129**. 97.

Leader. 1979. Manic states in affective disorders of childhood and adolescence. *Brit. Med. J.* **1**. 214.

Rutter, M. 1965. Classification and categorisation in child psychiatry. *J. Child Psychology and Psychiat.* **6**. 71.

Shaffer, D., Greenhill, L. 1979. A critical note on the predictive validity of 'the hyperkinetic syndrome'. *J. Child Psychology and Psychiat.* **20**. 61.

Wing, L. 1976. *Early Childhood Autism*. Pergamon. Oxford.

Index

abreaction, 77–84
acetycholine, 37
acting out, 159
aggression, 37, 39
alexithymia, 97
addiction, 143 *et seq.*
  amphetamines, 144–5, 160
  barbiturates, 144
  opiates, 143–4
alcohol, 4, 5, 48, 77–8, 149
alcoholism, 137, 143, 145–156
  voluntary organisations, 155
amphetamines, 144–5, 60
antidepressants, 5 *et seq.*, 51, 54, 136
  MAOI, 3, 4, 6, 7, 9, 11, 12, 18–25, 36, 39, 42, 45, 49, 53–4, 56, 82, 93, 100, 125, 129, 135, 139
    contraindications, 23
    interactions, 24
    iproniazid, 6
    isocarboxazid, 25
    Parstelin, 154
    phenelzine, 9, 19–22, 45, 135
    side effects, 22–3
    tranylcypromine, 9, 21, 22–25, 45, 125, 135, 139
  quadricyclics, 7
    maprotiline, 7, 9, 10, 11, 12, 16, 17–18
    mianserin, 8, 10, 11, 18
  tricyclics, 7 *et seq.*, 49, 82, 124, 126, 160
    overdosage, 14
    contraindications, 17
    amitriptyline, 3, 4, 7, 9, 10, 11, 12, 13, 14, 16, 133–4, 154
    butryptiline, 8, 10
    clomipramine, 7, 9, 10, 11, 16
    side effects, 14–16
    desipramine, 7, 8, 10
    imipramine, 3, 5, 6, 7, 9, 10, 16
    nortryptiline, 4, 8, 10, 11
    protryptiline, 8, 10
    side effects, 14–16
    trimipramine, 7, 8, 9, 10, 11, 14, 16, 135, 140, 154
  tricyclic-based drugs, 8
    dibenzepin, 8, 10
    dothiepin, 8, 10, 16, 139
    doxepin, 8, 10, 139
    nomifensine, 8, 10
  viloxazine, 8, 10
anorexia, 105 *et seq.*
anorexia nervosa, 36, 37, 39, 103 *et seq.*, 108–124
  body image, 111
  eating pattern, 108–9
  hunger and appetite, 109–110
  weight, 110
anxiety neurosis, 59, 84, 159
anxiolytics, 41 *et seq.*, 159
  diazepines, 44 *et seq.*, 129, 149, 154, 159–60
    contraindications, 47
    chlordiazepoxide, 1, 45
    clobazam, 46
    desmethyl diazepam, 44
    diazepam, 4, 44, 45, 46, 93, 135, 139, 149
    flurazepam, 46, 139, 141
    lorazepam, 44, 45, 46, 47, 149
    medazepam, 4, 46
    nitrazepam, 46, 139
    oxazepam, 44, 46, 47
    potassium chlorazepate, 46
    side-effects, 47
anti-Parkinsonian drugs, 3, 38–9, 41, 119
apomorphine, 152–3,

butyrophenones, 39–41
  benperidol, 41, 131
  droperidol, 41
  haloperidol, 33, 35, 40, 55, 139, 141, 149, 160
  triperidol, 41
behavioural psychotherapy, 42, 85–95, 124
  activity decrease, 90–91

activity increase, 89–90
activity loss, 91
activity acquisition, 88–9
aversion, 91, 151–2
aversion relief, 89–90
behavioural analysis, 87
biofeedback, 90, 94, 151
cognition change, 91–92
conditioning, 85
criticism of, 94–5
emotion change, 92–4
fading, 91
flooding, 93
graded exposure in vivo, 92
imaginal desensitisation, 92
implosion, 93
marital therapy, 89
motivation for change in, 88
rational emotive therapy, 91
response prevention, 91
role rehearsal/role reversal, 89
shaping, 85
social skills training, 88–9
targets, 87
token economy, 85

carbon dioxide, 83–4
cardiac neurosis, 21
catecholamines, 7
dopamine, 37, 40
noradrenaline, 7, 18, 23
childhood autism, 161–2
childhood psychosis, 159, 161
citrated calcium carbide, 153–4
coumarin anticoagulants, 43–4
cyproterone, 91, 131

delirium tremens, 44, 46, 149
dementia, 138, 140–2
depersonalisation, 58
depression, 3, 5, 7, 8, 13, 37, 52, 53, 54, 55, 56, 57, 84, 98, 100, 137, 138–140, 154, 159, 160–1
didrogesterone, 137
diethylpropion, 126
diphenylbutyl piperidines, 41
fluspirilene, 41
penfluridol, 41
pimozide, 41
Disablement resettlement officer, 33
disulfiram, 153–4

e.c.t., 1, 5–6, 7, 9, 10, 51–66, 100, 121, 140, 141, 161
anaesthesia for, 64–5
frequency of, 66
medico legal considerations of, 66
number of treatments, 63–4
risks and contraindications, 61–3
ether, 81

hallucinogens, 145
5-hydroxytryptamine, 7, 18, 23
hyperkinetic syndrome, 160
hypnosis, 81
hypnotics, 42, *et seq.,* 47–50
barbiturates, 43, 79–80, 160
barbitone, 43
butobarbitone, 43
methohexitone sodium, 65, 93
phenobarbitone, 43
quinal barbitone, 129
sodium amylobarbitone, 43, 56, 78, 79–80
thiopentone, 65
chloral hydrate, 48
chlormethiazole, 49, 141, 149
hypochondriasis, 58–9, 159
hysteria, 59

institutionalism, 1, 30
insulin, 1, 120
irritable bowel syndrome, 21–2

liothyronine, 18
lithium, 4, 5, 25–29, 35, 55, 124–5, 135–6, 138, 154
side effects, 27–29
toxicity, 29

mania, 35, 55
manic-depression, 26, 40, 53, 54, 137, 139
marihuana, 145
methylamphetamine, 78, 81, 82–3
methylphenidate, 160
myocardial infarction, 99–101

narcoanalysis, 77–84
nitrous oxide, 81

obesity, 124–6
obsessive-compulsive disorder, 16, 61, 84, 91, 158
occupational therapy, 1, 33
oestrogens, 131, 137

pain, 101–2
atypical facial, 21, 101
paraldehyde, 149
pharmacogenetics, 5
pharmacokinetics, 4
phenothiazines, 2, 4, 30 *et seq.,* 136, 160
side effects, 37–39
chlorpromazine, 1, 6, 11, 30, 31, 32, 35,

36, 37, 57, 107, 119–120, 124–5, 141, 160
fluphenazine, 33, 39
promazine, 160
thioridazine, 30, 31, 32, 37, 133, 141
trifluoperazine, 30, 33, 36, 133, 139, 141
phobic anxiety, 92, 93–5, 159
placebo effect, 2–3, 13, 44
post-natal 'blues', 134–5
pregnancy, 17, 29
'Premarin', 131, 137
premenstrual tension, 133, 136
progesterone, 4
propranolol, 45, 49–50
psychoanalysis, 81
psychophysiological symptoms, 20–21, 96 *et seq.*
psychosomatic medicine, 96–102
psychosurgery, 67–76, 121–2
conditions treated, 69
contraindications, 72
neuronal pathways, 69–72
procedures, 72–75
rehabilitation, 75–6
results, 68, 73–5
psychotherapy, 2, 42, 75, 77–84, 93, 95, 122–3, 155
puerperal psychosis, 132–6

reserpine, 1, 6, 139

schizo-affective disorder, 35, 57
schizophrenia, 26, 31–5, 40, 41, 50, 51, 52, 56–7, 84, 137
schizophreniform disorder, 35
sexual deviation, 129–131
sexual dysfunction, 127–9
sleep, 133
REM, 16, 47–9
non REM, 47–9
stupor
depressive, 61
schizophrenic, 61
suicide, 54, 75, 141

tardive dyskinesia, 38
testosterone, 128–9
therapeutic community, 1
thiamine, 150
thioxanthenes, 8, 33, 39
flupenthixol, 33, 39, 139, 141
thyrotropic hormone, 18
tics, 159
L-tryptophan, 18, 139

Weight Watchers, 126
Wernicke's encephalopathy, 150